Type II Diabetes and Your Health

Type II Diabetes and Your Health

Causes and Control—Plus Recipes to Aid Meal Planning

Helen V. Fisher

Introduction by Jeanette Parsons Egan, R.D.

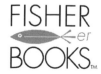

FISHER
BOOKS™

Library of Congress Cataloging-in-Publication Data
Fisher, Helen V.
      Type II diabetes and your health / Helen Fisher; introduction by
      Jeanette Egan.
         p. cm.
      Includes index.
      ISBN 1-55561-280-6
      1. Non-insulin-dependent diabetes—Popular works. 1. Title.
RC662.18. F55 2000
  616.4'62—dc2l

                             00-032165

Fisher Books is a member of the Perseus Books Group.

Find us on the World Wide Web at http://www.fisherbooks.com

Fisher Books titles are available at special discounts for bulk purchases in the United States by corporations, institutions and other organizations. For more information, please contact us.

Fisher Books
5225 W. Massingale Road
Tucson, Arizona 85743
(520) 744-6110

Text design by Anne Olson

First printing, October 2000

1 2 3 4 5 6 7 8 9 10-03 02 01 00

Contents

Introduction

Diabetes and Your Diet

Jeanette Parsons Egan, R.D.

What Is Diabetes?

Diabetes mellitus, usually called simply *diabetes* or formerly *sugar diabetes*, is a chronic condition in which the body does not produce any or enough insulin or cannot use it properly. The body's energy comes from the food we eat, which is broken down during digestion into glucose and other nutrients. Insulin is required to promote the movement of glucose into the cells. When it is lacking or insufficient, the body's cells cannot use glucose to provide energy, and the result is an accumulation of glucose in the blood. This excess blood glucose can lead to serious health problems (see "Complications Caused by Diabetes," page 8).

The American Diabetes Association (ADA) estimates that about 16 million people have diabetes, or about 5% of the population, in the United States. However, a disproportionate number of dollars, about 15%, is spent on medical care to treat diabetes. The Centers for Disease Control (CDC) lists diabetes as the seventh leading cause of death by disease in the United States. This ranking may be low, because deaths resulting from diabetes complications are believed to be underreported.

Types of Diabetes

There are three types of diabetes. Each type is different—having different causes and requiring different treatments—yet all are related to the way the body produces or uses insulin. Making the right food choices is an important factor in controlling each type.

Type I Diabetes

The first type of diabetes has been called *insulin dependent* because the pancreas produces little or no insulin. Therefore insulin must be injected several times each day. Diet and exercise are also important components of treatment. Five to 10% of people with diabetes have Type I. They usually develop diabetes at a young age, even as early as infancy, which is why Type I is also called *juvenile diabetes.*

Insulin

Insulin, a hormone that must be injected, remains the only, and essential, treatment for Type I diabetes. Insulin is not required for most people who have Type II diabetes, although many ask about it when they are first diagnosed. There are now several types of insulin available. Usually a person with Type I diabetes will inject insulin several times per day, using a combination of types. Some types work quickly and last only a few hours. Other kinds of insulin last longer and take longer to start working. Insulin is available in a premixed combination of short-acting and intermediate-acting insulin.

Type II Diabetes

Individuals with Type II diabetes produce insulin, but for some reason it does not function properly or they may not produce enough. Sometimes there is a lack of sufficient insulin receptors, reducing the amount of glucose that can enter the cells. In other cases the receptors do not operate correctly and are insulin resistant. Insulin resistance seems to be related to overweight. Persons with Type II diabetes usually control their condition with diet and exercise. If they are overweight, their doctor will usually recommend a calorie-controlled diet and exercise to encourage weight loss. Sometimes the doctor will prescribe oral medications (see "Oral Glucose-Lowering Agents," page 29) to reduce blood-glucose levels or, for people whose blood-glucose levels are very difficult to control, insulin.

Overweight, which is defined as a body mass index greater than 25 (see box, page 5), is a risk factor for developing Type II diabetes. People are usually diagnosed in middle age, which is why this type is sometimes called *adult-onset diabetes.* Recently, however, cases have been reported even in children and teenagers, perhaps because of the increasing incidence of overweight and physical inactivity among young people. One recent study has found that the prevalence of Type II diabetes has jumped by 70% from 1990 to 1998 among people between 30 and 39 years of age. People with a family history of diabetes and certain ethnic populations, particularly Native Americans, are also at risk.

Risk factors for developing Type II diabetes include

- Overweight
- Age 40 years or more
- Previous abnormal glucose test
- Family history of diabetes
- Member of an ethnic group with an increased risk for diabetes

---

Body Mass Index (BMI)

Body mass index is the ratio of a person's weight to his height and is only one of the values that dietitians use to evaluate nutrition status. People with above-average muscle mass may rate as overweight even though they're not.

To determine your BMI:
1. Divide your weight in pounds by 2.2
2. Divide your height in inches by 39.37
3. Multiply the number in Step 2 by itself
4. Divide the results of Step 1 by the results of Step 3. The resulting number equals body mass index.

Example:
1. 150 pounds ÷ 2.2 = 68.1
2. 65 inches ÷ 39.37 = 1.65
3. 1.65 x 1.65 = 2.72
4. 68.1 ÷ 2.72 = 25

Body Mass Index
Underweight: 19 or below
Healthy weight: 20 to 25
Overweight: 25 to 29.9
Obesity: 30 or above

Gestational Diabetes

Some women develop what is called *gestational diabetes* during pregnancy. This type of diabetes usually occurs in the later part of pregnancy when the woman's need for insulin increases as the baby grows. If the demand is not met, the mother becomes diabetic. Diet and exercise are usually the treatment of choice. If these do not bring glucose levels under control, insulin injections may be needed during the remainder of the pregnancy. Usually after the birth of the child, the mother's blood sugar levels return to normal, and insulin is no longer needed. However, women who have gestational diabetes are at risk of developing Type II diabetes later in life. Weight control after pregnancy is an important factor in preventing this outcome. Women who have had gestational diabetes should have their blood-glucose levels checked routinely.

Mothers with gestational diabetes tend to have larger babies because the high levels of glucose cause the baby's pancreas to produce more insulin. Because insulin is a growth stimulant, the baby gains weight more quickly. There is also an increased risk of a stillbirth.

Symptoms of Diabetes

Most cases of Type II diabetes are found during a routine physical examination that includes laboratory blood tests. Often there are few symptoms to alert the individual that he or she has diabetes. Anyone over the age of 40, especially if overweight or with a family history of diabetes, should have his or her blood-glucose levels checked.

Symptoms for Type II diabetes include
- Recurring skin, gum or bladder infections
- Frequent infections
- Slow healing of cuts and bruises
- Tingling or numbness in hands and feet
- Some of the same symptoms as Type I (below)
- Increased thirst
- No symptoms in some people

Because Type I diabetes has a more rapid onset, the symptoms are more extreme and urgent. They include
- Frequent urination
- Severe hunger and thirst
- Nausea and vomiting
- Sweet-smelling breath
- Fatigue
- Weight loss

Testing for Diabetes

According to the CDC, about one-third of the nearly 16 million people with diabetes are undiagnosed. The standard test for diabetes is a fasting plasma glucose test, which is usually taken after not eating for 12 hours. Two tests on separate days that result in a blood-glucose level greater than or equal to 126 mg/dL (milligrams per deciliter) confirm that an individual has diabetes. In individuals with symptoms of diabetes, two nonfasting blood-glucose levels greater than or equal to 200 mg/dL can confirm the diagnosis.

As many as 13 million people may have fasting glucose values of 110 to 125 mg/dL, just below the level for a diagnosis of diabetes. They are said to have *impaired fasting glucose.* Scientists are trying to determine how many of these people will later develop diabetes and what can be done to prevent it.

In response to the growing number of children and teenagers with Type II diabetes, the ADA's panel of experts issued the following recommendation in the March 2000 issue of *Pediatrics:*

> *There is no longer a special "diabetic" diet. The foods that people with diabetes eat are the same as those eaten by anyone who wants to consume a healthful diet.*

Children older than 10 years who weigh more than 120% of the ideal weight for their height should be tested for diabetes every two years if they have two other risk factors for diabetes.

Complications Caused by Diabetes

Untreated diabetes results in high levels of glucose (blood sugar) left in the blood with no way for the cells to use it for energy. These elevated levels of blood glucose can cause several serious side effects if they are not controlled. Complications include heart disease, stroke, blindness, impotence, kidney failure and loss of limbs due to infections caused by poor blood circulation. According to a 10-year study by the American Diabetes Association, complications from diabetes can be significantly reduced or delayed by controlling blood-glucose levels through self-monitoring, diet and medications. Keeping blood-glucose levels within normal values is important in controlling and preventing the complications (see box, below).

Complications in Persons with Diabetes, Compared to Those without Diabetes (CDC, 1998)

- Heart disease death rates 2 to 4 times higher
- Stroke risk 2 to 4 times higher
- Leading cause of blindness in persons 20 to 74 years old
- Higher incidence of gum disease, leading to tooth loss
- Increased risk of stillbirth
- Increased susceptibility to infectious diseases
- Some nervous system damage in about 65% of persons with diabetes
- High blood pressure in about 60% of persons with diabetes

Self-Monitoring Blood-Glucose Levels

Those with diabetes need to test their blood-glucose levels using a finger prick and testing strips. How often this is done depends on food intake, activity and medications. Follow the advice of your medical team. Keep accurate records, which will help the physician and dietitian evaluate your glucose control and make any necessary adjustments in treatment. For individuals with diabetes, glucose values before meals should probably be between 80 and 120 mg/dL, but check with your physician because everyone is different.

Symptoms of High Blood Sugar (Hyperglycemia)
(Usually more than 180 mg/dL)

- Nausea
- Thirst
- Frequent urination
- Tiredness
- Lightheadedness

Symptoms of Low Blood Sugar (Hypoglycemia)
(Usually less than 70 or 80 mg/dL)

- Dizziness
- Confusion or anger
- Sweaty or clammy skin
- Rapid heartbeat
- Fainting

Glycosylated Hemoglobin (HbAlc)

This is a test used to determine blood-glucose levels over a 3-month period. A laboratory must perform the test, and you may see it appear on a lab report. For individuals who do not keep a log of glucose values or keep incomplete records, this test is important in determining how well the diabetes is controlled. The results of the test give the health-care professional an indication of how well the

For most individuals with Type II diabetes, a well-planned, healthful diet with the appropriate calorie level is enough to control the disease.

person tested is controlling his or her glucose levels over a period of months, not just the day that blood is drawn to check blood glucose. This enables the health-care professional to make adjustments in medication or diet.

Controlling Diabetes through Diet

For most individuals with Type II diabetes, a well-planned, healthful diet with the appropriate calorie level is enough to control the disease. According to the ADA's Clinical Practice Recommendations 2000, the goals of nutrition therapy are

- Maintain near-normal blood-glucose levels
- Achieve optimal blood cholesterol and triglyceride levels
- Maintain or attain reasonable weight for adults
- Allow normal growth and development for children and teenagers
- Prevent and treat acute complications of insulin-treated diabetes
- Improve overall health

Dietary Recommendations

- 50 to 60% of total calories from carbohydrates
- 10 to 20% of total calories from protein
- About 30% of total calories from fat
- Less than 10% of total calories from saturated fat
- Less than 300 milligrams of cholesterol per day
- 20 to 35 grams of dietary fiber per day
- Less than 2000 to 2400 milligrams of sodium per day

There is no longer a special "diabetic" diet. The foods that diabetics eat are the same as those eaten by anyone who wants to consume a healthful diet. Foods should be low in saturated fat, high in fiber and good sources of vitamins and minerals. Calories should be controlled to achieve or maintain body weight within a reasonable range. The food intake for each

Teenagers and Children with Diabetes

Eating the same foods or foods that look the same as their peers is especially important for children and teenagers with diabetes so they do not appear "different." It really is easy to choose snacks and pack school lunches that feature their favorite foods and stay within recommended dietary guidelines. Because teenagers with Type II diabetes are usually overweight, careful planning of food intake is important. A dietitian can be very helpful in creating an eating plan that leads to weight loss and contains the nutrients that a teenager needs.

Always keep healthful snacks on hand for children and teenagers (see the Snacks chapter). This helps you to guide their food intake and prevents kids from turning to less healthful choices that may be higher in fat and empty calories.

If you have a child or teenager who is very active or takes part in organized sports, talk with a dietitian or certified diabetes educator about any changes that may need to be made in your child's diet.

diabetic should be determined in consultation with his or her health-care providers, usually a physician and a dietitian or diabetes educator, but the following are general guidelines.

Diabetes and Weight Control

Weight loss is important for those who have Type II diabetes and are overweight. Losing excess weight lowers insulin resistance, enabling the insulin to be used more efficiently. Weight loss of as little as 10 to 20 pounds can make a big difference in achieving glucose control. Often individuals with Type II diabetes on insulin or oral glucose-lowering drugs can quit taking medications after they reach a healthy weight and as long as they continue to maintain it.

Often individuals with Type II diabetes who are on insulin or oral glucose-lowering drugs can quit taking medications after they reach a healthy weight and as long as they continue to maintain it.

Other reasons to lose weight? All people with diabetes have a higher risk of heart disease. Losing weight lowers blood pressure, decreases cholesterol levels and improves circulation—all of which lowers the risk of heart disease.

Weight is best lost slowly, about one pound per week. Remember that it was probably gained slowly, and taking it off the same way will increase the likelihood that you will keep it off. Unfortunately, scientists have not discovered a safe "magic pill" for weight loss. Reducing calories and increasing activity are the ways to do it. (See "Diabetes and Exercise," page 25.)

Some Nutrition Basics

To learn how to choose foods wisely and plan your own meals, you need to understand a few facts about the nutrients that make up the different foods. With this knowledge, you will be better prepared to use the exchange lists (see page 217) and interpret the nutritional labels on the foods you buy.

Carbohydrates

Carbohydrates (starches and sugars), such as those from whole grains, fruits and vegetables, should provide the greatest percentage of calories, 50 to 60%. This is also the food group that supplies dietary fiber. No high-carbohydrate foods, including those containing sugar, are "forbidden" in the meal plans. The amount of carbohydrates eaten at meals and as snacks should be consistent each day, particularly for people on oral glucose-lowering medication or insulin. (To learn more about planning the number of starches to eat, read "Exchange Lists," page 19, and "Constant Carbohydrate Plan," page 20.)

Glycemic index. There is some evidence that certain carbohydrates increase the blood sugar more than others do, particularly in some people. This led to development of the glycemic index, which ranks carbohydrate foods according to how much the blood sugar increases in the two to three hours after eating. The higher the number, the more that the food is supposed to increase food glucose levels. For example, most dried beans are ranked low, whereas white bread and Cream of Wheat cereal are ranked much higher.

Even though there is a list ranking foods according to their glycemic index, it is not used very often in calculating carbohydrate intake or in teaching people with diabetes how to plan meals. For many people, the index is confusing to use. It ranks a limited number of foods. Also, some questions remain about its usefulness in helping people learn to control blood glucose. Bottom line: The total carbohydrate consumed is of more concern than the source of the carbohydrates.

Fats

The type as well as the amount of fat in the diet is important. Fats provide more than twice as many calories (9 calories per gram) as carbohydrates and protein, which have 4 calories per gram. A tip to remember if you're watching your weight: High-fat foods are high in calories. Fat should be limited to about 30% of total calories. The majority of it should be in monounsaturated form. Less than 10% of the calories should come from saturated fats, and less than 10% from polyunsaturated fats. Saturated fats can increase blood cholesterol levels, and monounsaturated fats tend to decrease blood cholesterol levels. Diabetes is a risk factor for developing heart disease, so a diet that contains fats that minimize that risk is important.

Hidden fats. Fats occur naturally in foods from animal sources, such as meats and dairy products, and in some plant sources, such as nuts, coconut and avocados. Fats are often hidden in prepared or packaged foods, such as baked goods,

Types of Fat

Monounsaturated Fats
   Canola oil
   Olive oil
   Olives
   Avocados
   Almonds
   Cashews
   Peanuts
   Peanut butter
   Pecans
   Sesame seeds

Polyunsaturated Fats
   Corn oil
   Margarine
   Safflower oil
   Soybean oil
   Sunflower seeds
   Walnuts

Saturated Fats
   Bacon
   Butter
   Cheese
   Coconut
   Cream
   Lard
   Palm oil
   Solid vegetable
      shortening

canned products and frozen meals. Often a low-fat or reduced-fat (or even fat-free) version of a commercial products exists. That's why it's so important to read food labels (see "Reading Food Labels," page 20).

Minimize fats when cooking. In addition, we add fat to foods during cooking or at the table— when we butter toast or put sour cream on a baked potato, for example. You can minimize fat consumption like this fairly easily. Use cooking spray, nonstick cookware and a minimum amount of fat in cooking food to reduce the amount of fat that you eat. When choosing margarine, look for one that has no more than 2 grams of saturated fat per tablespoon and has liquid oil as the first ingredient, not hydrogenated or partially hydrogenated oil.

Hydrogenation (adding hydrogen atoms) changes a liquid fat to a solid. In the process, the chemical makeup of the fatty acids changes from the *cis* to the *trans* form. Recent studies have shown that *trans* fatty acids increase LDL, the "bad," cholesterol levels, which is a risk factor for heart disease.

Read labels. Make it a habit to read labels to find out what kind of fat the food contains. The FDA has proposed changes in nutritional labeling that would require listing the amount of *trans* fatty acids in addition to the amount of saturated fat that is now listed. This hasn't happened yet, but it may be a change we will see in the near future.

Also look at the food itself for clues about hydrogenation. The softer the margarine, the fewer *trans* fatty acids that it contains, for example. The fat in natural peanut butter is less saturated than in regular peanut butter because it has not been hydrogenated to prevent it from separating when left at room temperature.

Finally, remember that fat in the diet is not "all bad." Some fat is necessary in the diet because it contains important nutrients, such as fat-soluble vitamins and essential fatty acids. Fat also adds flavor to foods and helps us feel satisfied after eating.

> ### Fat-Free and Reduced-Fat Foods
>
> Read the Nutrition Facts on the food label whenever you choose to buy a processed food product. Compare a fat-free product with a similar "regular" version. Sometimes the results will surprise you. Fat-free or reduced-fat does not mean "calorie-free." A fat-free or reduced-fat product may have about the same number of calories as the regular version. (Something—often sugar—has to be added to replace the fat.) Flavor is another factor that should affect your decision to buy. Would you rather have two very tasty cookies or four that are just okay? In general, reduced-fat products have better flavor and texture than fat-free products.

Protein

Protein should make up the remaining 15 to 20% of total calories. Good animal sources of protein are lean meats, poultry, seafood, low-fat dairy products and eggs. Most of the time, choose meats that have low to moderate amounts of fat—0 to 5 grams per ounce. Two to 3 ounces of cooked meat is usually enough for one adult serving.

Good vegetable sources of protein are dried beans, peas, lentils, tofu and peanut butter. Dried beans, peas and lentils are also good sources of fiber. Tofu is available in several versions, including seasoned and baked, and also in reduced-fat forms. Peanut butter is high in fat and so should be eaten in moderation. Starches and other vegetables have small amounts of protein; fruits have none.

Diabetes and the Family

A question new patients often ask, particularly women, is, "Do I have to prepare two meals—one for me and one for my family?" The answer is no. Foods that are included in the diabetic meal plans are healthful for the whole family to eat because they are generally lower in fat, calories and sugar and higher in fiber. There is an emphasis on vegetables, whole-grain breads and cereals and lean meats, but the foods can still be ones that are family favorites. Sometimes these recipes need modification to reduce the amounts or type of fat (particularly saturated fat) and calories.

Dietary Fiber—Two Kinds

Dietary fiber refers to the parts of plants that humans cannot digest. (Meat contains no fiber.) There are two kinds of fiber: soluble and insoluble. Usually both occur in the same foods. For example, apple skin is high in insoluble fiber, and the pulp of the apple is high in soluble fiber in the form of pectin. Sources of insoluble fiber include whole-grain cereals, wheat bran, seeds and fruit skins. Soluble fiber often forms a gel or gum when mixed with water. Sources of soluble fiber include dried beans and peas, apples, oat bran and rice bran.

Soluble fiber. Soluble fiber helps reduce blood cholesterol levels and controls the increase in blood glucose following a meal. Soluble fiber decreases both total blood cholesterol and low-density lipoprotein (LDL) cholesterol. High levels of LDL cholesterol are a risk factor for heart disease. Soluble fiber appears to work by reducing the reabsorption of cholesterol-containing bile acids from the small intestine. This cholesterol is then replaced from liver stores, reducing the amount in the body. Products formed during the fermentation of soluble fiber block the synthesis of cholesterol in the intestine, reducing the amount of cholesterol that is absorbed.

> *Soluble fiber helps reduce blood cholesterol levels and controls the increase in blood glucose following a meal. Insoluble fiber helps prevent constipation.*

Soluble fiber also helps to control blood-glucose levels after eating. It is thought that the fiber dissolves and slows stomach emptying, spreading the absorption of the glucose over a longer period of time.

Insoluble fiber. One of the most important functions of insoluble fiber is the prevention of constipation, because the fiber adds bulk and softness to the stool.

> *Adequate water intake is also important with a high-fiber diet—drink at last eight glasses of water each day, more if you are very active or live in a hot climate.*

Increase the amount of fiber in the diet slowly, over several weeks. This practice enables the digestive system to adapt and decreases problems that some individuals have with flatulence and abdominal cramps. Adequate water intake is also important with a high-fiber diet—drink at last eight glasses of water each day, more if you are very active or live in a hot climate.

To get an adequate amount of dietary fiber every day, the National Academy of Sciences recommends five or more servings of fruits and vegetables and six or more servings of whole-grain breads and cereals and dried beans and peas.

Sample Menu (about 1500 calories)

Breakfast
2-egg omelet with vegetables
2 slices whole-wheat toast with 2 teaspoons soft margarine
1 cup cantaloupe cubes
Coffee or tea

Snack
1 apple or other fruit

Lunch
2 cups vegetable soup   4 whole-wheat crackers
Mixed-green salad with tomatoes
2 to 3 tablespoons fat-free or low-fat salad dressing
8 ounces fat-free milk or soymilk

Snack
1 ounce sliced lean turkey   1 slice whole-wheat bread

Dinner
2 ounces grilled salmon
1/2 cup bulgur pilaf   1 cup cooked broccoli
1/2 cup cooked carrots   Sliced tomatoes or other raw vegetables
8 ounces fat-free milk or soymilk

Sample Menu (about 2000 calories)

Breakfast
1 cup cooked oatmeal with 1/4 cup chopped dried apricots
8 ounces fat-free milk
2 slices whole-wheat toast with 2 teaspoons soft margarine
1 cup orange slices
Coffee or tea

Snack
1 apple or other fruit   1 ounce reduced-fat cheese

Lunch
2 cups bean soup   4 whole-wheat crackers
Carrot sticks, celery sticks and radishes
2 to 3 tablespoons fat-free or low-fat salad dressing for dipping
8 ounces fat-free milk or soymilk

Snack
1 ounce sliced lean turkey   1 slice whole-wheat bread
1 tablespoon reduced-fat mayonnaise

Dinner
3 ounces lean roast beef or chicken
3/4 cup curried brown rice   1 cup cooked green beans
1/2 cup mashed sweet potatoes
Mixed greens and vegetable salad
2 to 3 tablespoons fat-free or low-fat salad dressing

Alcohol

Scientific research has established the benefits of moderate alcohol consumption, particularly wine, in lowering the risk of heart disease, which is prevalent among persons with diabetes. Because of these findings, people with diabetes who drink alcohol often ask about the place of alcohol in the diet. The position of the ADA is similar to the recommendation for all adults: Drink in moderation, one or two drinks per day. (But don't start drinking if you don't already do so, because for some people the risks of consuming alcohol are higher than the benefits.)

What's a Drink?
12 ounces beer
5 ounces wine
1½ ounces (80-proof) liquor

It is generally recommended that diabetics drink only if their blood-glucose levels are controlled and only with a meal or snack. This is especially important for Type I diabetics because drinking on an empty stomach can cause blood-glucose levels to decrease rapidly. In such cases, the person could appear drunk and not get the care that is needed in getting blood glucose back to normal levels.

If you are on oral glucose-lowering medications, always check with your physician before drinking because of possible drug interactions.

The calories in alcohol (7 calories per gram) are usually counted as fat or fat and starch exchanges; for example, a 12-ounce beer would equal 2 fat and 1 starch exchanges. For wine, dry is a better choice than sweet. Use unsweetened mixers when possible. Alcoholic beverages contain empty calories (that is, calories without nutrition), so beware if you're trying to lose weight.

Exchange Lists

One of the ways to calculate an individual eating plan is to follow the exchange lists that have been determined by the ADA and the American Dietetics Association (see Exchange

Lists, page 217). The exchanges are broken into groups of foods that have similar amounts of calories, carbohydrates, protein and fat. The groups are starches, fruits, milk, meats and meat substitutes, vegetables and fats. There are also lists of free foods and combination foods. If you think of the exchanges as servings, it is easy to determine a meal plan that can be individualized for each person's needs based on activity, caloric needs and insulin dosage or other medications. For example, in the vegetable group, each exchange (or serving), usually 1/2 cup, has 25 calories, 5 grams of carbohydrate, 2 grams of protein and 0 grams of fat. Starchy vegetables, such as potatoes, are grouped with the starches.

Constant Carbohydrate Plan

A more flexible approach to meal planning is just to count carbohydrates, consuming the same amount at the same time each day. Under this plan, starches, fruits and milk can be exchanged for each other because they each have about 15 grams of carbohydrate per serving. (Meats and fats contain no carbohydrates, and the vegetable group has very few.)

If you want to know more about using the exchange lists or carbohydrate counting to plan meals, talk with a registered dietitian or certified diabetes educator. Contact The American Dietetics Association at www.eatright.org or 800-877-1600, or the American Diabetes Association at www.diabetes.org or 800-342-2383 for more information.

Reading Food Labels

In 1990, Congress passed the Nutrition Labeling and Education Act, ensuring uniform and factual food labeling. Some items appearing on food labels because of this act are serving size, health claims and reference values for some nutrients, and definitions of such words as light and reduced-fat (see "Label Terms: What Do They Mean?" below). People with diabetes can use the Nutrition Facts on the label, particularly the amounts of carbohydrates and saturated fat, to determine how a specific food fits into their overall eating plan.

Label Terms: What Do They Mean?

When the terms *less, fewer* or *more* appear in nutrition claims, the referenced food does not have to be exactly the same as what it is being compared against. For example, one snack food might be compared to a different snack food, such as potato chips compared to pretzels. For the terms *light, reduced, added, extra, fortified* and *enriched* to be used, however, the foods must be similar—for example, light whole-wheat bread compared to regular whole-wheat bread.

Free (or "No")

- Calorie free: Less than 5 calories/serving
- Cholesterol free: Less than 2 milligrams cholesterol, 13 grams or less total fat, and 2 grams or less saturated fat
- Fat free: Less than 5 grams/serving
- Sodium free: Less than 5 milligrams/serving
- Sugar-free: Less than 5 grams/serving

Light

- Calories: 1/3 fewer calories than the standard product
- Fat: 50% of the fat of standard product
- Sodium: 50% less sodium, but must also be low calorie and low fat

---

Reduced or Less

- Reduced or less calories: 25% fewer calories than the standard product
- Reduced or less fat: 25% less fat compared to the standard product
- Reduced or less sodium: 25% less sodium compared to the standard product

more . . .

Low

- Low calorie: 40 calories or less/serving
- Low cholesterol: 20 milligrams or less cholesterol and 2 grams or less saturated fat/serving
- Low fat: 3 grams of fat or less/serving
- Low sodium: Less than 140 milligrams/serving
- Very low sodium: Less than 35 milligrams/serving

Lean and Extra Lean

These terms refer to meat, poultry, and seafood. Labels stating 5% fat refer to the percentage of fat by the weight of the product, not the percentage of calories from fat.

- Lean: Less than 10 grams total fat, less than 4 grams saturated fat, and less than 95 milligrams cholesterol per serving
- Extra lean: Less than 5 grams total fat, less than 2 grams saturated fat, and less than 95 milligrams cholesterol per serving

High and Good Source

These terms refer to the percentage of the Daily Value (DV), which is based on a 2,000-calorie daily intake, for a specific nutrient. For example, a food high in fiber (DV of 25 grams) would contain 5 grams or more of dietary fiber, whereas one that is a good source would have between 2.5 and 4.75 grams.

High: 20% or more of the DV per serving
Good Source: 10 to 19% of the DV per serving

No Sugar Added

No sugar or sugar-containing ingredients were added during processing. There may be natural sugars, and there must be a similar product available that does have added sugar. If it is not a low- or reduced-calorie product, the label must say so.

```
Nutrition Facts
Serving Size 1 Tbsp (14g)
Servings Per Container 32

Amount Per Serving
Calories 90     Calories from Fat 90

                           % Daily Value*
Total Fat  10g                      15%
  Saturated Fat 2g                  10%
  Polyunsaturated Fat 2.5g
  Monounsaturated Fat 2g
Cholesterol  0mg                     0%
Sodium 90mg                          4%
Total Carbohydrate  0g               0%
Protein  0g

Vitamin A                           10%
Not a significant source of dietary fiber,
sugars, vitamin C, calcium and iron.
*Percent Daily Values are based on a
 2,000 calorie diet.
```

INGREDIENTS: LIQUID SOYBEAN OIL AND PARTIALLY HYDROGENATED SOYBEAN OIL, WATER, WHEY, SALT, SOY LECITHIN, VEGETABLE MONO AND DIGLYCERIDES, POTASSIUM SORBATE AND CITRIC ACID AS PRESERVATIVES, ARTIFICIAL FLAVOR, COLORED WITH BETA CAROTENE, VITAMIN A (PALMITATE) ADDED.

Sample Nutrition Facts label.

Choosing Sweeteners

Sweeteners can be grouped as either caloric (containing calories) or noncaloric (fewer than 5 calories per serving). The caloric sweeteners include sugar (sucrose), fructose, corn syrup, honey, molasses and fruit juices.

Caloric Sweeteners

Sugar: No longer a no-no, sugar has been shown in studies not to raise blood-glucose levels any more than other carbohydrates, such as starches. But because many foods high in sugar are also high in fat and calories and low in important vitamins and minerals, these foods should be used in moderation as part of a balanced diet.

Fructose: Sometimes called *fruit sugar* because it is found in fruits and honey, fructose is sweeter than regular sugar (sucrose). Most recipes suggest using one-third less fructose than sucrose, which is made up of fructose and glucose. Fructose can be used for baking, but it is at its sweetest in chilled foods. Fructose may raise blood-glucose levels less than sucrose, but large amounts (greater than 20% of calories) can increase the levels of total cholesterol and LDL cholesterol. However, fructose can be used safely as a sweetener in moderation.

Mannitol, sorbitol and xylitol: These sugar alcohols have about half the calories of sugar but can act like a laxative and can cause cramping.

Other sweeteners: Corn syrup, honey, molasses, fruit juices and similar sweeteners can be used as part of the total carbohydrate in the diet in the same manner as sugar.

Noncaloric Sweeteners

Saccharin, aspartame, acesulfame-K and sucralose are the noncaloric sweeteners that have been approved for use by the FDA. They are generally recognized by the ADA as safe when used in moderation by persons with diabetes. Other sweeteners are under development and may be approved within the next few years.

Acesulfame-K: Two hundred times sweeter than sugar, this artificial sweetener was approved by the FDA in 1988. Stable in heat, it can be used for cooking, but it does have a bitter aftertaste when used in larger amounts. It is used commercially in beverages, puddings and syrups.

Aspartame: Known to consumers as *Equal* or *NutraSweet*, aspartame is about 200 times sweeter than sugar. The forms of aspartame available today cannot be used for cooking because heat destroys the sweetness. Use in cold foods and drinks.

Saccharin: Discovered in the late 1800s, saccharin is about 300 times sweeter than sugar. It has a bitter aftertaste that is intensified by heating.

Sucralose: Approved by the FDA in 1998 for use in commercial foods and as a table sweetener, sucralose is 600 times sweeter than sugar. It can be used for cooking because it is stable in heat. Sucralose is actually made from sugar but is not absorbed by the body. It is sold as *Splenda*.

Diabetes and Exercise

People with uncomplicated diabetes who have good glucose control can participate in most levels of activity. Trained athletes can even compete professionally. However, low blood sugar can occur during, immediately after, or hours after exercise. Anyone who wants to take part in strenuous exercise should be aware of the changes that exercise can cause. Self-monitoring of blood glucose is important so that adjustments in food and medications can be made as needed.

> *Exercise may help individuals with uncomplicated Type II diabetes maintain or achieve glucose balance by decreasing insulin resistance.*

Exercise may help individuals with uncomplicated Type II diabetes maintain or achieve glucose balance by decreasing insulin resistance. There is some disagreement as to the level and duration of exercise required to achieve this balance, but some studies have shown benefits from exercise as simple as brisk walking. Regular exercise can reduce triglyceride levels, reducing the risk of heart disease.

Physical activity is an important component of diabetes care, but those with diabetes or any chronic condition should always be evaluated by their physician before starting an exercise program. Patients with diabetes complications such as eye problems or loss of sensation in the feet may not be able to do more strenuous activities.

The Importance of Exercise

Exercise is one of the major components in blood sugar control for people with Type II diabetes. With both immediate and long-lasting benefits, exercise can

1. *Help with weight control.*

Exercise increases caloric expenditure, decreases appetite, and improves mood and self-esteem, helping you maintain or lose weight while you are watching caloric intake. It promotes long-term weight loss.

2. *Improve blood sugar control.*

Exercise decreases actual insulin resistance at the cellular level, plus it promotes weight loss, which further decreases insulin resistance. Cellular sensitivity to insulin happens during exercise and for several hours after exercise. Evening exercise, at least 1 1/2 to 2 hours after eating, tends to lower night and early-morning blood glucose levels.

3. *Improve the cardiovascular system and reduce diabetic complications.*

When muscles exercise or work, they can use three forms of energy, depending on the length and intensity of the workout: blood glucose; stores of glycogen (a starch), which can be changed into glucose when needed; and fat in the form of serum triglycerides. (When athletes use "carbohydrate loading" to increase endurance during an event, they are increasing their supply of glycogen.) The exercised muscle uses blood glucose first, then its own stored glycogen, and finally triglycerides to satisfy its need for energy. This reduces the amount of triglycerides in the arteries and veins. In addition, exercise can increase the level of HDL, or "good" cholesterol, and lower LDL, the "bad" cholesterol that glues cholesterol and triglycerides to the arteries and veins, clogging them and preventing blood flow. Exercise also reduces high levels of circulating insulin, which is a cardiovascular risk factor.

4. *Decrease blood pressure.*

By improving the fitness of the cardiorespiratory system— your heart, blood vessels and lungs—exercise may prevent strokes, heart attacks and poor circulation. Combined with a reduction in stress, exercise can lower blood pressure.

In addition to the above, exercise can strengthen your heart and lungs, increase your muscle tone and flexibility, improve digestion, decrease stress and anxiety and increase your energy and sense of well-being.

| **Silent Diabetes** |
| A friend who was recently diagnosed with Type II diabetes was shocked when his physician informed him that his blood-glucose level was over 180 mg/dL. As with many individuals without symptoms, his diabetes was found during a routine physical exam. He is now controlling his diabetes with weight loss, exercise and changes in the way he eats, mostly by reducing portion size. |

Guidelines for Designing an Exercise Program

Before you begin, see your doctor for a physical exam. Exercise can affect you in special ways that need to be evaluated. Once you are tested, you and your doctor can decide on the duration, type and intensity of your exercise program. When designing your personal exercise program, keep the following in mind:

1. Start with mild exercise for short periods of time. Gradually increase the time and intensity of your program.

2. To prolong insulin sensitivity and glucose utilization, exercise should be done 4 times a week or every other day.

3. For maximum continued weight reduction, exercise should be done 5 to 6 days a week.

4. Exercise should not cause shortness of breath. You should be able to talk during exercise, which is a better indicator of adequate pacing than taking your pulse.

5. Exercise should be limited in intensity so that your blood pressure does not rise above 180 mm Hg.

6. Aerobic exercise promotes cardiovascular fitness but should be low impact. Muscle-strengthening exercises are also recommended and can improve glucose utilization.

7. Warm-up and cool-down exercises are important to improve flexibility and prevent exercise-related injuries.

8. Fitness can be achieved in either of two ways:
    a. Exercising at 50 to 70% of predicted maximum heart rate for 20 minutes 4 to 7 days per week. Your doctor, dietitian or diabetes educator can help you determine what your maximum heart rate is and show you how to measure it.
    b. Participating in a physical activity at moderate intensity, such as a brisk walk or climbing stairs, for an accumulated 30 minutes or more each day.

Exercising Safely

1. Keep a form of diabetic identification (either a card or medallion) with you at all times.
2. Check your blood sugar before and after exercise.
3. Do warm-up and cool-down exercises to prevent injury.
4. Tell your exercise partner about your diabetes and explain what to do for hypoglycemic treatment.
5. Carry some form of real sugar, such as hard candy or glucose tablets.
6. Drink plenty of no-calorie liquids—water being the best.
7. Avoid extreme cold or hot temperatures. Exercise indoors during extreme weather.
8. Wear good-fitting shoes and check your feet for cuts, bruises or blisters after exercising. Treat any cuts or blisters promptly, and consult your physician if needed, because the feet of those with diabetes heal slowly and become infected easily.
9. Stop if you experience extreme discomfort or pain, lightheadedness, shortness of breath or nausea.

Pick the exercise for you, set realistic goals and have fun! By choosing a variety of activities or exercises, you will work various muscle groups and maintain your interest level. View your new exercise program as an opportunity to discover new activities, achieve new skills and make new friends. Your exercise program is another commitment to bettering your health—reducing stress, improving your self-esteem and simply feeling better.

Medications for Type II Diabetes

Proper meal planning and exercise, including weight loss, are the usual choices for controlling blood-glucose levels for those with Type II diabetes. However, if these measures are not enough, oral medications may be needed.

Oral Glucose-Lowering Agents

There are five classes of oral glucose-lowering medications prescribed for treating Type II diabetes. They are sometimes used in combination. Because the medications vary in their actions, your physician will prescribe one or more of them for you, depending on why your blood-glucose levels are high.

The classes and their mode of action are listed below. Of course, new medications to treat diabetes may be introduced that are not listed and some that are listed may be replaced by newer, safer and more effective ones. Always discuss your options with your doctor.

- *Sulfonylureas:* These drugs stimulate the pancreas to produce insulin. Medications include glipizide (Glucotrol), tolazamide (Tolinase), tolbutamide (Orinase) and glyuride (Diabeta).
- *Biguanide:* The only drug in this class, metformin hydrochloride (Glucophage), reduces the amount of glucose produced by the liver and decreases insulin resistance.
- *Alpha glucosidase inhibitors:* These delay the absorption of glucose from the small intestine into the blood. They include acarbose (Precose) and glyset (Miglitol).
- *Thiazolidinediones:* These drugs reduce the cells' resistance to insulin. They include pioglitazone hydrochloride (Actos) and rosiglitazone (Avandia).

- *Meglitinides:* This class is represented by only one drug, repaglinide (Prandin), which causes the pancreas to produce insulin in surges.

Diabetes Pills and Hypoglycemia

Everyone should understand that oral medications can cause hypoglycemia (low blood sugar) if an individual misses a meal or if the dosage needs to be adjusted. Hypoglycemia is not just a problem with those on insulin. Recently someone visiting my home asked if she could have a glass of orange juice. I could see that she was perspiring and starting to shake. She had taken her medication as usual but was too rushed to eat breakfast. The juice provided the glucose boost that she needed. Now she carries a sugary snack in case it happens again.

Insulin for Type-II Diabetics

As mentioned previously, insulin is sometimes prescribed for individuals with Type II diabetes who have difficulty achieving normal blood-glucose levels, either on a continuous basis or during periods of severe illness. Because of a long-term study showing the benefits of tighter blood-glucose control, in the future insulin may be prescribed more often for those with Type II diabetes.

Alternative Medicines

As in other areas of medical care, several herbs have been suggested as alternative treatments for Type II diabetes. Some of these are in the process of being tested for effectiveness and safety. Before taking herbs, discuss them with your health-care professionals, because herbs can interact with prescribed medications. Remember that herbs can have potential adverse side effects. Just because they are natural doesn't mean that they are safe.

Easy-to-Prepare Recipes for Living Well with Type II Diabetes

Appetizers

The first course can be called an appetizer, a starter, or an antipasto—whatever the name, the purpose is the same; that is, to whet your appetite with a little bit of food before dinner. Because this is the beginning of your meal, think in terms of small portions. You don't want these tidbits to be too rich or filling.

Offer your guests foods or snacks that will complement the meal to come. It's best to serve more than one item because you can't expect everyone to like your one choice. Eye appeal is important; be sure you make an inviting presentation. Choose foods that contrast one another in taste, texture, and color; for example, a creamy-smooth seafood dip accompanied by crunchy raw vegetables. Fancy foods are not necessary; a bowl of nuts, along with crackers and cheese slices, can be elegant. People with diabetes in particular should try to include protein of some kind.

I like to allow at least 30 minutes to one hour to linger with guests before serving the main meal. This is a welcoming time, especially for those people who are meeting for the first time.

Most of all, relax and enjoy your own party!

Avocado-Caper Spread

Pistachios add texture as well as flavor to this delicate avocado spread.

1/2 medium avocado, peeled
1/2 cup (115 g) nonfat cream cheese
1 teaspoon grated lemon zest
2 teaspoons lemon juice
2 tablespoons chopped pistachios
2 teaspoons chopped fresh cilantro
2 teaspoons capers

Mash avocado and cream cheese together until blended; stir in remaining ingredients. Serve on toasted bagels or pita bread triangles. Makes 1 cup.

Each tablespoon contains:

Cal.	Cal. from Fat	Protein	Carb.	Total Fiber	Total Fat	Sat. Fat	Chol.	Sodium
24	13	2g	1g	0g	1g	0g	1mg	51mg

Exchanges:

1/2 Fat

Broccoli Flowers

Create attractive, flowerlike bundles for your next buffet or picnic.

    1 pound (450 g) fresh broccoli crowns
    3 tablespoons crumbled herbed feta cheese
    1 tablespoon nonfat mayonnaise
    1 tablespoon plain nonfat yogurt
    1/2 teaspoon Dijon-style mustard
    1 (5-ounce/140-g) package very thinly sliced cooked chicken
        (about 20 slices)

Trim broccoli; cut flowers and stems into about 18 pieces 3 to 4 inches (7.5 to 10 cm) long. Steam in a 2-quart (2-liter) saucepan about 5 minutes or until tender; drain. Combine feta cheese, mayonnaise, yogurt, and mustard. Spread one side of each chicken slice with mayonnaise mixture. Place one piece of cooked broccoli in center of each slice. Roll up like a cornucopia with broccoli flower protruding through the open end. Serve warm or cold. Makes 6 servings.

Each serving contains:

Cal.	Cal. from Fat	Protein	Carb.	Total Fiber	Total Fat	Sat. Fat	Chol.	Sodium
63	15	8g	5g	2g	2g	1g	14mg	451mg

Exchanges:

1 Lean Meat/Protein, 1 Vegetable, 1/2 Fat

Bruschetta

Enliven Italian bread with fragrant olive oil and your favorite herbs.

6 slices Italian or French bread
1 garlic clove, minced
1 tablespoon chopped fresh basil or
    1 teaspoon dried leaf basil
1 tablespoon chopped fresh parsley
1/2 teaspoon dried leaf oregano
2 tablespoons olive oil
1/2 teaspoon garlic powder
1 teaspoon crushed anise seeds

Place bread slices on baking sheet. Preheat broiler or toaster oven. In a small bowl, thoroughly combine remaining ingredients until well blended. Brush each slice of bread with mixture. Place under broiler and brown; turn slices and brush again. Return to broiler. Toast until brown. Serve at once. Makes 6 servings.

Each serving contains:

Cal.	Cal. from Fat	Protein	Carb.	Total Fiber	Total Fat	Sat. Fat	Chol.	Sodium
124	51	3g	15g	1g	6g	1g	0mg	176mg

Exchanges:

1 Bread/Starch, 1 Fat

Caponata

Serve this eggplant and tomato classic as a cold relish or dip.

2 tablespoons olive oil
1 small eggplant, cut into small cubes
1 onion, chopped
1 garlic clove, minced
2 celery stalks, chopped
1/4 cup (28 g) thin strips dry-pack sun-dried tomatoes
2 fresh tomatoes, chopped
1 green or yellow bell pepper, seeded and chopped
1/4 cup (30 g) pitted green olives
1 cup (250 ml) no-salt-added tomato juice
1/4 cup (60 ml) red wine vinegar
2 tablespoons chopped fresh parsley

In a large nonstick skillet, heat oil. Add eggplant; sauté 2 or 3 minutes. Stir in onion, garlic, celery, sun-dried tomatoes, fresh tomatoes, bell pepper, olives, tomato juice, and wine vinegar. Simmer 10 to 15 minutes, stirring occasionally, until vegetables are tender. Stir in parsley. Cool. Spoon into a serving bowl, cover and refrigerate until chilled. Serve on lettuce leaves as a first course or with crackers as a dip. Makes 48 servings (3 cups).

Each tablespoon contains:

Cal.	Cal. from Fat	Protein	Carb.	Total Fiber	Total Fat	Sat. Fat	Chol.	Sodium
12	6	0g	2g	0g	1g	0g	0mg	23mg

Exchanges:

Free

Chicken Quesadilla

A filling Mexican appetizer that can also be served for a light lunch.

4 (8- to 10-inch/20- to 25-cm) flour tortillas
1/2 cup (55 g) shredded Monterey Jack cheese
1 cup (170 g) chopped cooked chicken
1/4 cup (30 g) chopped green onions, including tops
2 tomatoes, seeded and chopped
2 roasted green chiles, peeled, seeded, and chopped
1 to 2 tablespoons chopped fresh cilantro
Shredded lettuce
4 tablespoons fat-free sour cream
1/2 avocado, peeled and chopped
1/2 cup (115 g) tomato salsa

On one half of each tortilla, distribute cheese, chicken, green onions, tomatoes, green chiles, and cilantro. Fold plain half over fillings, making a half moon shape. Place in a medium nonstick skillet and cook over medium heat until underside is lightly browned. Turn tortilla over and brown other side; cheese should be melted. Slide onto serving plate and slice into wedges. Place a small amount of lettuce next to folded edge and garnish with sour cream, avocado, and salsa. Makes 8 appetizer servings.

Each wedge contains:

Cal.	Cal. from Fat	Protein	Carb.	Total Fiber	Total Fat	Sat. Fat	Chol.	Sodium
177	63	10g	19g	1g	7g	2g	22mg	248mg

Exchanges:

1 Bread/Starch, 1 Very Lean Meat/Protein, 1 Vegetable, 1 1/2 Fat

Barbecue Chicken Bites

Spear pieces of chicken from a zesty sauce.

1/2 cup (115 g) canned jellied cranberry sauce
1 (8-ounce/230-g) can unsweetened crushed pineapple,
   drained
1/2 teaspoon grated fresh ginger
1/2 cup (115 g) thick hickory-smoke barbecue sauce
3 cups (500 g) cubed cooked chicken

In a 2-quart (2-liter) nonstick saucepan, combine cranberry sauce, pineapple, ginger, and barbecue sauce. Stir over low heat until cranberry sauce dissolves. Add chicken and continue cooking until hot. Have wooden picks handy for serving. Makes about 45 chicken pieces.

Each piece contains:

Cal.	Cal. from Fat	Protein	Carb.	Total Fiber	Total Fat	Sat. Fat	Chol.	Sodium
27	7	3g	2g	0g	1g	0g	8mg	32mg

Exchanges:

1/2 Very Lean Meat/Protein

Olive-Stuffed Meatballs

A tasty treat lies inside these little gems.

1/2 pound (230 g) extra-lean ground beef
1 green onion, chopped
1/4 cup (20 g) quick-cooking rolled oats
1 egg white
2 teaspoons chopped capers
1/2 teaspoon dried leaf basil
1/2 teaspoon dried leaf marjoram
1 tablespoon chopped fresh parsley
1 tablespoon low-sodium tomato sauce
Black pepper to taste
20 pimiento-stuffed olives

In a small mixing bowl, combine beef, green onion, oatmeal, egg white, capers, basil, marjoram, parsley, tomato sauce, and pepper. Thoroughly mix ingredients. Take a scant tablespoonful of meat mixture and pat into a patty; press an olive in center. Pinch meat around olive. Repeat with remaining olives. Place in a large nonstick skillet. Cook until browned on all sides. Cover and cook 5 minutes more. Makes 20 meatballs.

Each tablespoon contains:

Cal.	Cal. from Fat	Protein	Carb.	Total Fiber	Total Fat	Sat. Fat	Chol.	Sodium
29	14	3g	1g	0g	2g	0g	4mg	103mg

Exchanges:

1/2 Lean Meat/Protein

Oregano-Flavored Chips

What could be easier than adding extra flavor to a familiar snack?

4 corn tortillas
1 egg white
1 teaspoon dried leaf oregano
1 teaspoon mild chili powder

Preheat oven to 425F (220C). Line a baking sheet with foil.
Cut tortillas in half, then into wedges. Spread tortillas in one
layer on prepared baking sheet. Whisk egg white until frothy;
add oregano and chili powder. Whip to blend. Brush each
tortilla wedge with mixture. Bake until lightly browned, 5 to
6 minutes. Makes 4 servings.

Each serving contains:

Cal.	Cal. from Fat	Protein	Carb.	Total Fiber	Total Fat	Sat. Fat	Chol.	Sodium
65	7	2g	13g	2g	1g	0g	0mg	62mg

Exchanges:

1 Bread/Starch

Shrimp Spread

Especially good on raw vegetables, as well as crackers or toasted bagels.

3 ounces (85 g) cooked shrimp, chopped
1/4 cup (55 g) nonfat cream cheese
2 tablespoons plain nonfat yogurt
2 tablespoons nonfat cottage cheese
2 teaspoons lemon juice
2 tablespoons chopped pimiento
3 tablespoons capers
1 teaspoon prepared horseradish
1 green onion, chopped
Dill weed to taste

In a small bowl, blend shrimp, cream cheese, yogurt, cottage cheese, and lemon juice. Stir in remaining ingredients. Cover and refrigerate until ready to serve. Serve with toasted pita wedges or crackers. Makes 16 servings (1 cup).

Each tablespoon contains:

Cal.	Cal. from Fat	Protein	Carb.	Total Fiber	Total Fat	Sat. Fat	Chol.	Sodium
12	1	2g	1g	0g	0g	0g	8mg	90mg

Exchanges:

Free

Sun-Dried Tomato Dip

The Mediterranean flavors of this dip pair well with toasted pita bread wedges.

1/2 cup (115 g) low-fat cottage cheese
1/2 cup (115 g) nonfat cream cheese
3 oil-packed sun-dried tomatoes, chopped
2 tablespoons lemon juice or vinegar
1 tablespoon chopped fresh basil or parsley
2 green onions, chopped
1/2 teaspoon dry mustard
2 teaspoons chopped capers
1 teaspoon caper juice
1/4 cup (30 g) chopped red bell pepper

In a bowl, combine all ingredients. Pour into 2-cup (1-pint) serving container; cover and refrigerate several hours before serving. Makes 20 servings (1/ cups).

Each tablespoon contains:

Cal.	Cal. from Fat	Protein	Carb.	Total Fiber	Total Fat	Sat. Fat	Chol.	Sodium
12	1	2g	1g	0g	0g	0g	1mg	106mg

Exchanges:

Free

Yakitori Chicken Kabobs

Mirin can be found in the Asian food section of your supermarket.

Yakitori Sauce:
1/4 cup (60 ml) mirin (sweet rice wine)
2 tablespoons reduced-sodium soy sauce
1½ teaspoons grated fresh ginger
1 green onion, chopped
1 garlic clove, minced
1/4 teaspoon sesame oil

3/4 pound (340 g) skinned and boned chicken, cut into 1-inch (2.5-cm) cubes

In a medium mixing bowl, combine yakitori sauce ingredients. Add cubed chicken and marinate at least 30 minutes. Preheat broiler. Thread chicken cubes on skewers. Broil 5 to 7 minutes, turning and brushing with marinade several times during cooking. Makes 4 servings.

Each serving contains:

Cal.	Cal. from Fat	Protein	Carb.	Total Fiber	Total Fat	Sat. Fat	Chol.	Sodium
159	43	18g	6g	0g	5g	1g	54mg	353mg

Exchanges:

2½ Very Lean Meat/Protein, 1½ Fat

Soups

Homemade soup brings back memories of home and tasty, nourishing, simple meals. Homemade soup is what I grew up with; it wasn't until I was a teenager that I tasted canned soups. They didn't—couldn't—compare to my mother's soups.

In today's busy world, we always seem to be looking for the winning combination of something that is easy to fix, can be prepared ahead and will be well received by all. Soup is the answer. For something out of the ordinary, serve Butternut Squash & Apple Soup or Artichoke Bisque. Albóndigas, a Mexican soup, is an example of a complete meal in a bowl. If this one is new to you, be adventuresome and try it.

Cold soups are the perfect antidotes to warm weather. Think of them as a salad you can spoon. I like to serve a chilled soup, such as Cold Zucchini Soup, on the patio. To keep it cold on a warm day, place the serving bowl within a larger bowl filled with ice. Set out a tray with garnishes, cups and a ladle for stirring and serving. Let guests serve and garnish their own bowls.

Warming cream soups can help turn a small portion of leftovers, usually vegetables, into a satisfying dish. Served in a cup as a starter or in a bowl as the main course, soup is welcome at any meal. In fact, in some Middle European and Far Eastern countries, soup is even served for breakfast, a pleasant and nutritious way to start the day.

Making a vegetable broth that vegetarians will enjoy is truly simple. Basically it is flavored water, made by simmering vegetables and herbs or spices. I much prefer using this to plain water. Start with 4 quarts water and one cup each chopped carrots, celery and onion. If you like, add other vegetables and dried seasoning such as bay leaf. Simmer about 1 hour. I feel fresh herbs yield more flavor if they are added during the last 5 minutes of cooking. Don't overlook using lots of fresh parsley— luckily, it's always available. Strain and discard the vegetables and refrigerate or freeze in small containers until needed.

Artichoke Bisque

A different combination of subtle flavors.

1 tablespoon olive oil
1/2 cup (55 g) chopped onion
1 tomato, chopped
1 cup (80 g) sliced fresh mushrooms
1 (10-ounce/280-g) package frozen artichokes, thawed
    and chopped
1 cup (250 ml) low-sodium chicken broth
1 cup (250 ml) water
1/2 cup (55 g) frozen green peas
3 tablespoons all-purpose flour
1 tablespoon cornstarch
2 cups (500 ml) evaporated skimmed milk
Salt and black pepper to taste

In a 3-quart (3-liter) nonstick saucepan, heat oil and sauté onion until softened, not browned. Add tomato, mushrooms, artichokes, broth and water. Cook about 5 minutes or until tender. Add peas. Blend flour and cornstarch with evaporated milk; add to soup and cook 5 to 7 minutes or until slightly thickened. Season with salt and pepper. Makes 5 (1-cup) servings.

Each serving contains:

Cal.	Cal. from Fat	Protein	Carb.	Total Fiber	Total Fat	Sat. Fat	Chol.	Sodium
185	34	12g	27g	4g	4g	1g	4mg	175mg

Exchanges:

1/2 Bread/Starch, 1½ Vegetable, 1 Skim Milk, 1/2 Fat

Albóndigas

A traditional Mexican soup of meatballs in a tomato broth, made with chicken rather than beef.

1/2 pound (230 g) skinned and boned chicken, ground
1/4 onion, chopped
1 egg white
1/4 cup (22 g) quick-cooking rice
4 cups (1 liter) low-sodium chicken broth
6 cups (1.5 liters) water
1/4 cup (60 ml) low-sodium tomato sauce
2 roasted green chiles, peeled, seeded and chopped
1 fresh tomato, chopped
1 carrot, julienned
2 green onions, cut into 2-inch (5-cm) lengths
1/4 teaspoon dried leaf oregano
1/3 cup (55 g) frozen corn kernels
2 tablespoons chopped fresh cilantro

In a small bowl, combine chicken, onion, egg white and rice. Using about 1 tablespoon for each, form mixture into 1-inch (2.5-cm) balls. Set aside. In a 5 1/2-quart (5.5-liter) nonstick Dutch oven, combine broth, water, tomato sauce, chiles, tomato, carrot, green onions, oregano and corn. Bring mixture to a boil. Add meatballs, reduce heat, and simmer about 30 minutes. Add cilantro and cook 5 minutes more. Serve hot. Makes 10 (1-cup) servings.

Each serving contains:

Cal.	Cal. from Fat	Protein	Carb.	Total Fiber	Total Fat	Sat. Fat	Chol.	Sodium
69	15	7g	7g	1g	2g	1g	15mg	53mg

Exchanges:

1/2 Bread/Starch, 1 Very Lean Meat/Protein, 1/2 Vegetable

Beef Barley Soup

Sweet potatoes bring a different taste to this hearty dish.

1 pound (450 g) boneless short ribs or beef shank, cubed
3 cups (750 ml) low-sodium beef broth
3 cups (750 ml) water
1 onion, chopped
1 cup (140 g) chopped peeled sweet potato
2 celery stalks, chopped
3 tomatoes, chopped
1/2 teaspoon ground cumin
1/3 cup (55 g) pearl barley
2 tablespoons chopped fresh parsley
Salt and black pepper to taste

Brown beef cubes in a 5-quart (5-liter) nonstick Dutch oven over medium heat. Add broth, cover, and cook 25 minutes. Add remaining ingredients. Cover and simmer about 1 hour or until barley and vegetables are tender. Makes 6 to 8 (1-cup) servings.

Each serving contains:

Cal.	Cal. from Fat	Protein	Carb.	Total Fiber	Total Fat	Sat. Fat	Chol.	Sodium
267	94	21g	22g	4g	10g	4g	48mg	92mg

Exchanges:

1 Bread/Starch, 3 Very Lean Meat/Protein, 1 Vegetable, 2 Fat

Butternut Squash & Apple Soup

A pretty soup that combines two fall favorites, apples and squash.

1/2 cup (55 g) chopped roasted yellow or orange bell pepper
2 pounds (900 g) butternut squash, peeled, seeded and
cut into 1-inch (2.5-cm) pieces
1/2 cup (115 g) chopped onion
2 green apples (340 g), peeled and chopped (2 cups)
2 cups (500 ml) low-sodium chicken broth
1 cup (250 ml) unsweetened apple juice
1 cup (250 ml) water
1 teaspoon grated fresh ginger
1/4 teaspoon ground mace
1/4 teaspoon ground nutmeg
2 tablespoons chopped toasted almonds, for garnish

In a large pot, combine all ingredients except almonds. Cover
and cook until vegetables are tender. Purée mixture in batches
in a food processor or blender. Reheat and serve garnished
with almonds. Makes 8 (1-cup) servings.

Each serving contains:

Cal.	Cal. from Fat	Protein	Carb.	Total Fiber	Total Fat	Sat. Fat	Chol.	Sodium
102	16	2g	22g	4g	2g	0g	1mg	34mg

Exchanges:

1 Bread/Starch, 1/2 Fruit, 1/2 Vegetable, 1/2 Fat

Chicken Tortilla Soup

Here is an innovative use for leftover chicken. The tortillas can be a little stale too.

2 teaspoons olive oil
3 green onions, chopped
1 garlic clove, minced
1 tomato, seeded and chopped
4 cups (1 liter) chicken broth
1 cup (170 g) shredded cooked chicken
2 roasted green chiles, peeled, seeded and chopped
1 cup (250 ml) water
2 corn tortillas, cut into strips
1/2 cup (55 g) shredded low-sodium, low-fat Monterey
    Jack cheese
1 avocado, peeled, pitted and sliced

Heat oil in a 3-quart (3-liter) saucepan and sauté green onions and garlic until softened, not browned. Add tomato, broth, chicken, chiles and water. Simmer, uncovered, about 15 minutes. Preheat oven to 325F (165C). Place tortilla strips on a baking sheet and bake 7 to 10 minutes or until lightly browned. Remove and place strips and cheese in bottom of each serving bowl. Ladle soup into bowls and garnish with avocado slices. Makes 6 servings.

Each serving contains:

Cal.	Cal. from Fat	Protein	Carb.	Total Fiber	Total Fat	Sat. Fat	Chol.	Sodium
182	98	12g	10g	3g	11g	2g	27mg	122mg

Exchanges:

1/2 Bread/Starch, 1 1/2 Very Lean Meat/Protein, 1/2 Vegetable, 2 Fat

Chinese Vegetable Soup

Chicken and pork make a flavorful combination.

1 tablespoon vegetable oil
1 tablespoon grated fresh ginger
1 chicken thigh, skinned, boned and chopped
1/2 pound (230 g) cubed fat-trimmed pork tenderloin
3 cups (750 ml) low-sodium chicken broth
3 cups (750 ml) water
3 green onions, chopped
1 (8½-ounce/245-g) can sliced water chestnuts, drained
1/4 pound (115 g) fresh mushrooms, sliced
1/4 pound (115 g) fresh bean sprouts, rinsed and drained
1/2 cup (55 g) frozen green peas
2 teaspoons reduced-sodium soy sauce
Salt and black pepper to taste

Heat oil and ginger in a 5½-quart (5.5-liter) nonstick Dutch oven. Add chicken and pork; lightly brown. Add broth, water and green onions; bring to a full boil. Reduce heat and simmer 20 minutes. Add water chestnuts and mushrooms. Continue cooking 5 minutes or until mushrooms are tender. Add bean sprouts and peas; cover and cook 2 to 3 minutes. Stir in soy sauce. Season with salt and pepper. Serve at once. Makes 12 (1-cup) servings.

Each serving contains:

Cal.	Cal. from Fat	Protein	Carb.	Total Fiber	Total Fat	Sat. Fat	Chol.	Sodium
76	28	7g	5g	1g	3g	1g	17mg	78mg

Exchanges:

1 Very Lean Meat/Protein, 1 Vegetable, 1/2 Fat

Confetti Corn Chowder

Bright colors and flavors abound in this chowder.

2 bacon strips, chopped
2 green onions, including tops, chopped
1 celery stalk, chopped
2 (14-ounce/400-g) cans low-sodium cream-style corn
1 tablespoon chopped pimiento
1 cup (250 ml) low-sodium chicken broth or water
1 1/2 cups (375 ml) low-fat milk
1 tablespoon chopped fresh tarragon or
    1 teaspoon dried tarragon
Salt and black pepper to taste

Sauté bacon in a 3-quart (3-liter) nonstick saucepan. Stir in green onions and celery. Add remaining ingredients except salt and pepper and simmer, uncovered, 15 to 20 minutes. Season with salt and pepper. Makes 6 (1-cup) servings.

Each serving contains:

Cal.	Cal. from Fat	Protein	Carb.	Total Fiber	Total Fat	Sat. Fat	Chol.	Sodium
171	52	6g	28g	2g	6g	2g	8mg	488mg

Exchanges:

1 1/2 Bread/Starch, 1/2 Skim Milk, 1 Fat

Minestrone Soup

Warm and satisfying, a meal that is ideal for a cold day.

1 tablespoon olive oil
1 onion, chopped
2 celery stalks, chopped
2 carrots, sliced
1 small zucchini, sliced
1/2 cup (125 g) canned garbanzo beans (chickpeas)
1 (8-ounce/230-g) can no-salt-added tomatoes with juice
2 bay leaves
1/2 teaspoon dried Italian seasoning
1 cup (250 ml) low-sodium beef broth
1 cup (250 ml) no-salt-added tomato juice
5 cups (1.25 l) water
1 tablespoon chopped fresh parsley
2 cups (85 g) chopped fresh spinach
1 ounce (28 g) small shells, cooked

In a 5½-quart (5.5-liter) nonstick Dutch oven, heat oil. Sauté onion, celery and carrots. Add zucchini, garbanzo beans, tomatoes with juice, bay leaves, dried Italian seasonings, broth, tomato juice and water. Bring to a boil, reduce heat, and cook over medium heat until vegetables are tender, about 30 minutes. Add parsley, spinach and pasta. Cook another 2 to 3 minutes. Remove and discard bay leaves. Makes 8 (1-cup) servings.

Each serving contains:

Cal.	Cal. from Fat	Protein	Carb.	Total Fiber	Total Fat	Sat. Fat	Chol.	Sodium
80	21	3g	13g	3g	2g	0g	0mg	87mg

Exchanges:

1/2 Bread/Starch, 1 Vegetable, 1/2 Fat

Cream of Mushroom Soup

For an interesting appearance and slightly different flavor, combine different types of mushrooms.

1 pound (450 g) fresh mushrooms
1 tablespoon margarine
2 cups (500 ml) homemade vegetable broth (see page 45)
2 cups (500 ml) water
1/2 teaspoon dried leaf basil
2 cups (500 ml) evaporated skimmed milk
2 tablespoons flour
1 tablespoon cornstarch
1/4 cup (60 ml) dry white wine
Salt and black pepper to taste

Rub mushrooms with a damp paper towel. Trim mushrooms and slice or chop them in small pieces. In a 3-quart (3-liter) nonstick saucepan, melt margarine; add mushrooms. Stirring frequently, cook mushrooms until lightly browned. Add broth, water and basil. Heat to boiling; simmer gently 30 minutes. Remove pan from heat. Blend evaporated milk and flour together; add to mixture. Return pan to heat; stir and simmer until soup thickens. Add wine. Do not allow soup to boil again. Season with salt and pepper. Serve hot. Makes 6 (1-cup) servings.

Each serving contains:

Cal.	Cal. from Fat	Protein	Carb.	Total Fiber	Total Fat	Sat. Fat	Chol.	Sodium
123	22	8g	17g	1g	2g	1g	3mg	107mg

Exchanges:

1 Vegetable, 1 Skim Milk, 1/2 Fat

Creamed Spinach-Rice Soup

Add more curry powder if you like food a bit spicier.

1 tablespoon olive oil
1/2 onion, chopped
1/2 cup (85 g) chopped cooked chicken
4 cups (1 l) low-sodium chicken broth
2 cups (500 ml) water
1/4 cup (22 g) long-grain white rice
1/2 teaspoon curry powder
1/4 teaspoon ground nutmeg
1 1/2 cups (375 ml) evaporated skimmed milk
3 tablespoons all-purpose flour
1/2 (10-ounce/280-g) package frozen spinach
Salt and black pepper to taste

Heat oil in a 5-quart (5-liter) nonstick Dutch oven. Sauté onion and add chicken, chicken broth, water, rice, curry powder and nutmeg. Cover and reduce heat; simmer 20 to 25 minutes. In a small bowl, blend evaporated milk and flour. Stir into soup mixture, add spinach, and cook until slightly thickened. Season with salt and pepper. Makes 6 to 8 (1-cup) servings.

Each serving contains:

Cal.	Cal. from Fat	Protein	Carb.	Total Fiber	Total Fat	Sat. Fat	Chol.	Sodium
154	38	11g	18g	1g	4g	1g	15mg	159mg

Exchanges:

1/2 Bread/Starch, 1 Lean Meat/Protein, 1/2 Vegetable, 1/2 Skim Milk, 1/2 Fat

Tomato-Lentil Soup

There's wholesome goodness in every satisfying spoonful.

1 cup (170 g) dried lentils
1/2 onion, chopped
1 carrot, sliced
1 celery stalk, sliced
1 red bell pepper, seeded and sliced
1/2 teaspoon ground cinnamon
1/2 teaspoon ground cardamom
1/2 teaspoon black pepper
4 cups (1 l) homemade vegetable broth (see page 45) or water
1 (16-ounce/450-g) can tomatoes
1 (10-ounce/280-g) package frozen broccoli spears
Salt to taste

Rinse and sort lentils. In a 5½-quart (5.5-liter) nonstick Dutch oven, combine lentils, onion, carrot, celery, bell pepper, cinnamon, cardamom, black pepper and broth. Bring to a boil. Cover, reduce heat, and simmer about 30 minutes or until lentils are done. Add tomatoes and broccoli; cook until tender. Season with salt. Serve hot. Makes 8 (1-cup) servings.

Each serving contains:

Cal.	Cal. from Fat	Protein	Carb.	Total Fiber	Total Fat	Sat. Fat	Chol.	Sodium
58	2	4g	11g	4g	0g	0g	0mg	108mg

Exchanges:

1/2 Bread/Starch, 1 Vegetable

Roasted Tomato & Red Pepper Soup

For a creamier soup, purée all of the mixture.

4 red bell peppers, halved and seeded
2 Roma tomatoes, halved and seeded
1 tablespoon olive oil
1/2 small onion, chopped
1 celery stalk, chopped
1 garlic clove, minced
2 cups (500 ml) low-sodium chicken broth or fat-free milk
2 tablespoons cornstarch
1/2 cup (120 ml) water
2 tablespoons chopped fresh chives or green onion tops,
    for garnish

Preheat broiler. Place bell peppers and tomato halves, cut side down, on a broiler rack. Broil until skin blisters evenly, turning with tongs if needed. Cool slightly and scrape off skin. Coarsely chop peppers and tomatoes.

In a large saucepan, heat oil and sauté onion, celery and garlic. Add peppers and tomatoes and cook about 2 minutes. Add chicken broth or milk, reduce heat, and simmer about 15 minutes. Dissolve cornstarch in water; slowly pour into tomato mixture. Stirring constantly, cook until thickened.

Remove from heat and cool slightly. Purée about one-fourth of mixture in a food processor or blender and return to pan. Blend together and heat. Serve at once, garnished with chopped chives. Makes 6 (1-cup) servings.

Each serving contains:

Cal.	Cal. from Fat	Protein	Carb.	Total Fiber	Total Fat	Sat. Fat	Chol.	Sodium
74	27	2g	11g	2g	3g	1g	1mg	47mg

Exchanges:

2 Vegetable, 1/2 Fat

Vegetarian Vegetable Soup

This soup is especially good with warm cornbread.

4 cups (1 l) homemade vegetable broth (see page 45)
1 bay leaf
1/2 teaspoon dill weed
Pinch of black pepper
1½ cups (215 g) diced potatoes
1/2 cup (55 g) diced onion
3 carrots, sliced 1/4 inch (6 mm) thick
2 cups (230 g) sliced zucchini
2 tomatoes, chopped
1/2 cup (85 g) frozen lima beans
Salt to taste

Combine broth, bay leaf, dill weed, pepper, potatoes, onion and carrots in a 2-quart (2-liter) nonstick saucepan. Bring mixture to a full boil, partially cover, reduce heat, and simmer 20 minutes. Add zucchini, tomatoes and lima beans; cook 10 minutes longer or until all vegetables are tender. Season with salt. Serve hot. Makes 6 (1-cup) servings.

Each serving contains:

Cal.	Cal. from Fat	Protein	Carb.	Total Fiber	Total Fat	Sat. Fat	Chol.	Sodium
82	3	3g	18g	4g	0g	0g	0mg	32mg

Exchanges:

1 Bread/Starch, 1 Vegetable

Cold Zucchini Soup

Cold soups make a refreshing change on a warm day.

3 medium zucchini
1 cup (250 ml) low-sodium chicken broth
1 cup (250 ml) water
1/2 teaspoon dill weed
1/8 teaspoon garlic powder
1 cup (230 g) plain nonfat yogurt
1 cup (250 ml) evaporated skimmed milk
Raw zucchini or 2 tablespoons chopped pimiento, for garnish
2 tablespoons chopped fresh parsley, for garnish
Sprinkle of paprika
Salt and black pepper to taste

Wash zucchini and cut into 1/4-inch-thick (6-mm-thick) slices. Place zucchini, broth, water, dill weed and garlic powder in a 2-quart (2-liter) nonstick saucepan. Bring to a boil, reduce heat, and simmer 5 minutes or until zucchini is tender. Remove from heat and cool. Pour mixture into a blender or food processor. Add yogurt and evaporated milk and purée. Refrigerate several hours. Serve cold with garnish of fresh zucchini slices or pimiento, parsley and a sprinkle of paprika. Season with salt and pepper. Makes 6 (1-cup) servings.

Each serving contains:

Cal.	Cal. from Fat	Protein	Carb.	Total Fiber	Total Fat	Sat. Fat	Chol.	Sodium
70	4	7g	11g	1g	0g	0g	3mg	95mg

Exchanges:

1/2 Bread/Starch, 1/2 Skim Milk

Salads

Salads can be served as the appetizer, main dish, or side dish of a meal or as a palate cleanser after the entrée. However you serve it, be certain to include at least one salad in your meal plans every day.

When making a mixed green salad, select some of the new greens that are available. They have subtle differences in flavor, and some have vibrant color differences. For more robust flavor, use romaine or try chicory (curly endive), which is even stronger—almost pungent. Do not confuse it with Belgian endive, an almost white, small, slender head that is pleasantly bitter. For added interest, include contrasting colors such as red leaf lettuce or the beautiful radicchio (Italian chicory), which has white veins contrasting with deep red leaves.

Garnishing is that extra touch that is noticed and welcomed by all, so save your prettiest sprig of fresh herbs for a place of honor when presenting the salad. Or dazzle guests with a garnish of edible flowers, such as nasturtiums, borage flowers, squash blossoms, pansies, rose petals and pot marigold (calendula), which will transform your salad into a spectacular dish.

Main-dish salads are particularly welcome during the warm summer months. Celebrate the brief season when cherries are plentiful by making a hearty Chicken Cherry Salad. Monterey Chicken Salad is a colorful and filling main dish that contains my favorite Mexican ingredients. Serve Greek Salad or Turkey-Peach Salad along with a crusty French bread for a wonderful meal on the patio.

Kidney Bean Salad

A wonderful way to use leftover beans.

1 cup (230 g) cooked kidney beans, drained
1/2 cup (115 g) canned yellow soybeans, rinsed and drained
1/2 cup (55 g) corn kernels, cooked and drained
1 zucchini, sliced
1 green onion, chopped
1 tomato, chopped
1/4 pound (115 g) jícama, peeled and cut into sticks
1 tablespoon lemon juice
1 bunch fresh spinach or mixed salad greens
1 tablespoon chopped fresh parsley

Combine kidney beans soybeans, corn, zucchini, green onion, tomato, jícama and lemon juice. Place in a covered container and refrigerate about 1 hour or until well chilled. Rinse spinach or mixed salad greens and pat dry. Line salad plates with spinach or greens. Spoon bean mixture over spinach, dividing evenly, and sprinkle with parsley. Makes 6 servings.

Each serving contains:

Cal.	Cal. from Fat	Protein	Carb.	Total Fiber	Total Fat	Sat. Fat	Chol.	Sodium
100	17	7g	16g	6g	2g	0g	0mg	30mg

Exchanges:

1 Bread/Starch, 1/2 Lean Meat/Protein, 1/2 Vegetable

Cabbage & Carrot Slaw

A dash of color and flavor makes this an eye-appealing salad.

1/4 cup (60 ml) cider vinegar
1/4 cup (60 ml) vegetable oil
1 teaspoon sugar
1 teaspoon dry mustard
1/2 teaspoon celery seed
1 teaspoon grated onion
1 teaspoon salt
4 cups (340 g) shredded green cabbage
1 carrot, shredded
1 medium orange, peeled and cut into small chunks

In a 1-quart (1-liter) nonstick saucepan, combine vinegar, oil, sugar, dry mustard, celery seed, onion and salt. Stir over medium heat until sugar dissolves. Cool to room temperature. Combine cabbage, carrot and orange in a large bowl. Pour dressing over; toss to coat. Makes 6 to 7 servings.

Each serving contains:

Cal.	Cal. from Fat	Protein	Carb.	Total Fiber	Total Fat	Sat. Fat	Chol.	Sodium
111	83	1g	8g	2g	9g	1g	0mg	400mg

Exchanges:

1 Vegetable, 2 Fat

Red Cabbage Slaw

Dress our colorful picnic slaw with Balsamic Herb Dressing, page 80.

3 cups (260 g) shredded red cabbage
2 celery stalks, sliced
1/4 cup (30 g) corn kernels, cooked and drained
1/2 cup (85 g) green seedless grapes
1 apple, cored and sliced
1/2 cup (85 g) dried currants

In a salad bowl, mix cabbage, celery, corn, grapes, apple and currants. Toss with dressing. Makes 6 servings.

Each serving (without dressing) contains:

Cal.	Cal. from Fat	Protein	Carb.	Total Fiber	Total Fat	Sat. Fat	Chol.	Sodium
74	3	1g	19g	3g	0g	0g	0mg	17mg

Exchanges:

1 Fruit, 1/2 Vegetable

Chicken Cherry Salad

A cool, light, main-dish salad. To avoid staining your hands when pitting fresh cherries, wear latex or thin rubber gloves or place your hands inside a large plastic food bag and use as gloves. Serve with crusty bread and a cold drink.

1 cup (170 g) cubed cooked chicken
1/2 cup (75 g) pitted fresh Bing cherries
1/2 cup (85 g) green seedless grapes
1 apple, cored and sliced
1 cucumber, peeled and sliced
1/2 cantaloupe, peeled and cubed
1/4 head lettuce, torn into bite-size pieces
Yogurt-Cucumber Dressing, page 85

Chill all ingredients. Combine in a large bowl and toss with dressing. Spoon onto serving plates. Makes 4 servings.

Each serving (without dressing) contains:

Cal.	Cal. from Fat	Protein	Carb.	Total Fiber	Total Fat	Sat. Fat	Chol.	Sodium
149	30	12g	20g	3g	3g	1g	31mg	39mg

Exchanges:

1½ Very Lean Meat/Protein, 1 Fruit, 1 Vegetable, 1/2 Fat

Monterey Chicken Salad

A surprising combination of fruit, vegetables and citrus vinaigrette elevates this chicken salad from the ordinary.

3/4 cup (170 g) cooked black beans, drained
1/2 cup (60 g) chopped peeled jícama
1/3 cup (40 g) green peas, cooked
2 tablespoons chopped pimiento
3/4 cup (130 g) cubed cooked chicken
1 banana, sliced
3 tablespoons orange juice
2 tablespoons canola oil
1 tablespoon chopped fresh cilantro
1 green onion, chopped
Salt and black pepper to taste
Lettuce

Chill all ingredients. In a large mixing bowl, combine beans, jícama, peas, pimiento, chicken and banana. In a cup, stir together orange juice, oil, cilantro and green onion. Pour over bean mixture. Gently toss. Season with salt and pepper. Line a serving dish with lettuce leaves; top with bean mixture. Serve at once. Makes 6 servings.

Each serving contains:

Cal.	Cal. from Fat	Protein	Carb.	Total Fiber	Total Fat	Sat. Fat	Chol.	Sodium
138	55	8g	14g	3g	6g	1g	16mg	18mg

Exchanges:

1/2 Bread/Starch, 1 Very Lean Meat/Protein, 1/2 Fruit, 1/2 Vegetable, 1 Fat

Couscous Fruit Salad

If you haven't tried couscous, you'll find it quick to prepare. Combine it with tropical fruits and spices for a hearty salad that can be served warm or cold.

1⁄ cups (300 ml) pineapple-orange juice
1/4 teaspoon ground cinnamon
1/4 teaspoon ground mace
1 cup (185 g) couscous
1 cup (200 g) drained canned pineapple chunks
1 banana, sliced
2 teaspoons lemon juice
1/2 avocado, peeled, pitted and chopped
3 tablespoons chopped almonds, toasted

Place pineapple-orange juice, cinnamon and mace in a 1-quart (1-liter) nonstick saucepan; heat until boiling. Stir in couscous. Cover and remove from heat. Let stand 5 minutes. Spoon in pineapple chunks. Pour mixture into a serving bowl. Top with banana slices. Sprinkle banana slices with lemon juice. Top with avocado and almonds. Makes 6 servings.

Each serving contains:

Cal.	Cal. from Fat	Protein	Carb.	Total Fiber	Total Fat	Sat. Fat	Chol.	Sodium
142	47	3g	23g	3g	5g	1g	0mg	5mg

Exchanges:

1/2 Bread/Starch, 1 Fruit, 1 Fat

Cucumber-Tomato Salad

Pretty layers of red and green are topped by the crunch of sunflower seeds. Try zucchini in place of the cucumber.

1 cucumber, thinly sliced

1 red onion, thinly sliced

2 tomatoes, thinly sliced

2 tablespoons olive oil

1 tablespoon wine vinegar or apple cider

2 tablespoons lemon juice

1/4 teaspoon garlic powder

1/4 teaspoon dill weed

1 tablespoon chopped fresh basil or

    1 teaspoon dried leaf basil

2 teaspoons unsalted sunflower seeds, toasted

In a salad bowl, alternate slices of cucumber, red onion and tomatoes. In a cup, blend oil, vinegar or cider, lemon juice, garlic powder, dill weed and basil. Pour over cucumber mixture and sprinkle with sunflower seeds. Cover and chill before serving. Makes 4 to 6 servings.

Each serving contains:

Cal.	Cal. from Fat	Protein	Carb.	Total Fiber	Total Fat	Sat. Fat	Chol.	Sodium
103	70	2g	8g	2g	8g	1g	0mg	10mg

Exchanges:

1½ Vegetable, 1½ Fat

Crab and Shrimp Salad

Mango complements the fresh flavors of two seafood favorites.

Lettuce or spinach leaves
1 mango, peeled, pitted and sliced
1/2 cup (115 g) cooked small shrimp
1/2 cup (115 g) cooked crab
2 celery stalks, sliced
1 green onion, finely chopped
1 cucumber, sliced
12 cherry tomatoes
2 limes or lemons

Line 4 plates with lettuce or spinach leaves. Place one-fourth of mango slices on each plate. Combine shrimp and crab and mound on top of mango; top with celery and green onion. Place cucumber slices and cherry tomatoes on the side. Cut limes or lemons into wedges; place on plates. Let each person squeeze wedges over salad as desired. Makes 4 servings.

Each serving contains:

Cal.	Cal. from Fat	Protein	Carb.	Total Fiber	Total Fat	Sat. Fat	Chol.	Sodium
111	16	11g	15g	3g	2g	0g	69mg	170mg

Exchanges:

1 1/2 Very Lean Meat/Protein, 1/2 Fruit, 1 1/2 Vegetable

Green Bean & Potato Salad

With its unexpected combination of ingredients, this is no ordinary potato salad. Top with Italian Dressing, page 83.

2 cups (300 g) green beans, cooked
1 cup (85 g) sliced fresh mushrooms
2 cups (450 g) sliced peeled cooked potatoes
1/2 cup (55 g) chopped celery
3 green onions, chopped
1/4 red bell pepper, seeded and chopped
1/4 cup (30 g) raisins
1/4 cup (30 g) corn kernels, cooked
2 tablespoons chopped capers
2 tablespoons pine nuts

In a large salad bowl, combine all ingredients. Cover and refrigerate at least 4 hours. Add dressing before serving. Makes 6 servings.

Each serving (without dressing) contains:

Cal.	Cal. from Fat	Protein	Carb.	Total Fiber	Total Fat	Sat. Fat	Chol.	Sodium
100	15	3g	21g	3g	2g	0g	0mg	104mg

Exchanges:

1/2 Bread/Starch, 1/2 Fruit, 1 Vegetable, 1/2 Fat

Greek Salad

Serve with crusty French bread. The Greeks dip the bread into the dressing rather than butter it.

3 tomatoes, chopped
2 cucumbers, sliced
1/2 green bell pepper, seeded and sliced
1/2 onion, chopped
4 radishes, sliced
1 tablespoon chopped capers
1/2 teaspoon dried leaf oregano
2 tablespoons wine vinegar
2 tablespoons olive oil
Lettuce leaves, torn into bite-size pieces
1 ounce (30 g) feta cheese, crumbled
12 black Greek olives

In a large bowl, combine tomatoes, cucumbers, bell pepper, onion and radishes. Mix together capers, oregano, vinegar and oil. Pour over mixture and toss. Chill before serving. Spoon mixture onto lettuce leaves, top with cheese and garnish with olives. Serve with crusty French bread. Makes 4 servings.

Each serving contains:

Cal.	Cal. from Fat	Protein	Carb.	Total Fiber	Total Fat	Sat. Fat	Chol.	Sodium
145	92	4g	12g	3g	10g	2g	6mg	405mg

Exchanges:

2 1/2 Vegetable, 2 Fat

Mixed Green Salad

Try one of the prepackaged salad combinations that contains greens of contrasting colors, textures and flavors.

6 cups (300 g) mixed salad greens, torn into bite-size pieces
1 celery stalk, sliced
1/2 green bell pepper, seeded and sliced
1/2 sweet red onion, thinly sliced
1 tablespoon chopped fresh herbs, such as parsley, basil and cilantro
2 to 3 tablespoons French Dressing, page 81

In a bowl, toss greens, celery and bell pepper, onion and fresh herbs together. Add dressing and toss again to coat. Makes 6 servings.

Each serving contains:

Cal.	Cal. from Fat	Protein	Carb.	Total Fiber	Total Fat	Sat. Fat	Chol.	Sodium
43	8	2g	6g	2g	2g	0g	0mg	47mg

Exchanges:

1 Vegetable, 1/2 Fat

Old-Fashioned Potato Salad

A yogurt dressing gives this familiar salad extra tang.

3 cups (12 ounces) cooked new potatoes
1/4 cup (30 g) chopped celery
2 tablespoons chopped green olives
1/2 cup (55 g) green peas, cooked
1/4 cup (30 g) chopped green onion
1/2 teaspoon chopped fresh dill
1 tablespoon chopped fresh parsley
2 tablespoons lemon juice
2 tablespoons nonfat mayonnaise
1/3 cup (85 g) plain nonfat yogurt
2 tablespoons chopped fresh chives
Black pepper to taste
1 sprig fresh dill, for garnish

Slice potatoes and place in a large bowl. Add remaining ingredients except dill sprig; toss gently to combine. Garnish with dill sprig. Serve warm or cold. Makes 4 servings.

Each serving contains:

Cal.	Cal. from Fat	Protein	Carb.	Total Fiber	Total Fat	Sat. Fat	Chol.	Sodium
142	6	4g	31g	4g	1g	0g	0mg	161mg

Exchanges:

1½ Bread/Starch, 1/2 Vegetable

Mediterranean Salad

Cooking spray provides an easy way to add just a touch of oil to your salad.

1 large tomato, seeded and diced
1 large green bell pepper, seeded and diced
1 large cucumber, seeded and diced
6 radishes, diced
12 pitted small green olives
1 tablespoon chopped fresh parsley
2 teaspoons red wine vinegar
1/2 teaspoon black pepper
Bibb lettuce

Combine tomato, bell pepper, cucumber, radishes, olives and parsley in a large bowl. Spray with olive oil cooking spray. Mix well. Sprinkle vegetables with vinegar and black pepper. Toss well. Chill about 1 hour. Serve over lettuce leaves. Makes 6 servings.

Each serving contains:

Cal.	Cal. from Fat	Protein	Carb.	Total Fiber	Total Fat	Sat. Fat	Chol.	Sodium
31	11	1g	5g	1g	1g	0g	0mg	193mg

Exchanges:

1 Vegetable

Pear-Grapefruit Salad

Make this winter salad when grapefruit come to market and apples and pears are still at their peak.

Lettuce or spinach leaves
1 pear, cored, peeled and sliced
1 red grapefruit, peeled and cut into segments
1 apple, cored and cut in eighths
1/2 cup (85 g) red seedless grapes
2 tablespoons chopped pecans
4 teaspoons balsamic vinegar

Arrange lettuce or spinach leaves on 4 salad plates. Top with alternating slices of pear, grapefruit and apple. Top with grapes and pecans. Drizzle with vinegar. Makes 4 servings.

Each serving contains:

Cal.	Cal. from Fat	Protein	Carb.	Total Fiber	Total Fat	Sat. Fat	Chol.	Sodium
124	26	1g	26g	6g	3g	0g	0mg	3mg

Exchanges:

1½ Fruit, 1/2 Fat

Three Bell-Pepper Salad

You can enjoy wonderful color as well as flavor with this great salad. If desired, top with a spoonful of dressing.

1 cup (230 g) canned black soybeans, rinsed and drained
1 red bell pepper, seeded and julienned
1 yellow or orange bell pepper, seeded and julienned
1 green bell pepper, seeded and julienned
2 green onions, chopped
1 cup (85 g) sliced fresh mushrooms
1 tablespoon chopped fresh basil or
     1 teaspoon dried leaf basil
Spinach or romaine lettuce leaves
1 tablespoon pumpkin seeds, toasted

In a bowl, toss together all ingredients except spinach leaves and pumpkin seeds. Line salad plates with spinach or romaine lettuce leaves. Place bell pepper mixture on top of leaves. Sprinkle with pumpkin seeds. Makes 4 to 6 servings.

Each serving contains:

Cal.	Cal. from Fat	Protein	Carb.	Total Fiber	Total Fat	Sat. Fat	Chol.	Sodium
81	11	6g	12g	5g	1g	0g	0mg	4mg

Exchanges:

1/2 Bread/Starch, 1/2 Very Lean Meat/Protein, 1 1/2 Vegetable

Ricotta-Melon Salad

Treat yourself to a cool, satisfying luncheon salad that doesn't need a dressing.

1 cantaloupe
1 cup (230 g) reduced-fat ricotta cheese
1/4 cup (60 ml) orange juice
1 banana, sliced
2 kiwis, peeled and sliced
16 blueberries

Peel melon, cut in half, and remove seeds; cut into slices. Divide slices equally among 4 plates. In a small bowl, stir ricotta and orange juice together. Fold in banana slices. Mound ricotta mixture on top of melon slices. Arrange kiwi slices attractively around sides. Top ricotta mound with blueberries. Makes 4 servings.

Each serving contains:

Cal.	Cal. from Fat	Protein	Carb.	Total Fiber	Total Fat	Sat. Fat	Chol.	Sodium
196	50	9g	30g	3g	6g	3g	19mg	92mg

Exchanges:

1 Lean Meat/Protein, 2 Fruit, 1/2 Fat

Turkey-Peach Salad

Fresh berries make a pretty as well as tasty addition.

1 bunch fresh spinach
1 cup (170 g) cubed cooked turkey
1 celery stalk, sliced
2 fresh peaches, peeled, pitted and sliced
1 cup (140 g) fresh raspberries or strawberries
2 tablespoons chopped pecans, toasted
2 tablespoons House Salad Dressing (page 82)

Thoroughly rinse spinach. Pat dry and tear into bite-size pieces. In a salad bowl, combine spinach, turkey, celery, peaches, berries and pecans. Toss gently with dressing. Or line 6 salad plates with spinach; arrange celery, turkey and peaches on top. Scatter berries on top and drizzle with dressing. Sprinkle with pecans. Makes 6 servings.

Each serving contains:

Cal.	Cal. from Fat	Protein	Carb.	Total Fiber	Total Fat	Sat. Fat	Chol.	Sodium
102	40	8g	8g	3g	4g	1g	18mg	45mg

Exchanges:

1 Very Lean Meat/Protein, 1/2 Fruit, 1/2 Fat

Dressings, Salsas & Sauces

While a salad or entrée may be complete in itself, often the addition of a complementary dressing, salsa or sauce gives it a special taste that makes it memorable. That's what this chapter is all about.

While I choose a light-flavored oil for most cooking, I will reach for a more robust olive oil when I feel it will enhance the flavor of a dish or dressing. Walnut and avocado oils make wonderful salad dressings, as well.

Enhance a simple vinaigrette by making your own flavored vinegars. This requires some forethought because the best results come after the flavors have been allowed to blend at least three weeks. Experiment with both herb and fruit combinations. A few minutes' preparation can result in a dressing that has your personal touch.

The chipotle chile may be new to you. This brown, plump chile has a distinctive smoky flavor. Canned chipotle chiles can be found in the specialty or Mexican food section of your market. Dried varieties can be purchased in produce markets featuring Hispanic ingredients.

Flavorful salsas can turn plain broiled chicken, fish, or meat into a festive entrée. Served as a side dish, they brighten any meal, and at our house we especially enjoy them with sandwiches. For ease of preparation, try my uncooked Papaya-Pineapple Salsa, which can also be made with other fruits, such as mango, peach, apricot or pear.

When introducing spicy salsas, serve small portions alongside foods. Don't serve on top of food until you've tasted it. Fruit-based salsas such as Cantaloupe Salsa or Papaya Salsa contain a small amount of green chile; add more if you like. The combinations can surprise the palate.

Balsamic Herb Dressing

A simple dressing that features the special deep, rich flavor of balsamic vinegar.

3 tablespoons balsamic vinegar
2 tablespoons lemon juice
6 tablespoons olive oil
3 garlic cloves, crushed
1/2 teaspoon dry mustard
1/2 teaspoon dried leaf basil
1/2 teaspoon dried leaf oregano
1/2 teaspoon paprika

Combine all ingredients in a jar with a tight-fitting lid. Or blend ingredients in a food processor or blender. Store in a covered container. Shake salad dressing vigorously before using. Makes about 2/3 cup (160 ml).

Each tablespoon contains:

Cal.	Cal. from Fat	Protein	Carb.	Total Fiber	Total Fat	Sat. Fat	Chol.	Sodium
75	73	0g	1g	0g	8g	1g	0mg	1mg

Exchanges:

1½ Fat

French Dressing

My favorite dressing for a mixed green or vegetable salad.

1/2 cup (120 ml) olive oil
1/4 cup (60 ml) cider vinegar
2 tablespoons grated onion
1/3 cup (85 g) low-sodium catsup
1 teaspoon paprika
1 teaspoon black pepper
1 tablespoon lemon juice
1/2 teaspoon Dijon-style mustard
2 garlic cloves

Place all ingredients in a blender and mix well. Pour into a container and cover. Chill before using. Garlic cloves can remain in dressing or removed. Shake vigorously before pouring on salad greens. Makes about 1/ cups (300 ml).

Each tablespoon contains:

Cal.	Cal. from Fat	Protein	Carb.	Total Fiber	Total Fat	Sat. Fat	Chol.	Sodium
54	49	0g	2g	0g	5g	1g	0mg	52mg

Exchanges:

1 Fat

House Salad Dressing

Use this recipe as a marinade for cooked vegetables.

1/3 cup (80 ml) olive oil
1/4 cup (60 ml) cider vinegar
1/2 teaspoon dried leaf basil
1/2 teaspoon dried leaf marjoram
1 teaspoon dry mustard
1/2 teaspoon paprika
1/2 teaspoon Worcestershire sauce
1 garlic clove, chopped

Combine all ingredients. Let stand at room temperature at least 2 hours. Stir vigorously before using. Makes about 2/3 cup (160 ml).

Each tablespoon contains:

Cal.	Cal. from Fat	Protein	Carb.	Total Fiber	Total Fat	Sat. Fat	Chol.	Sodium
66	65	0g	1g	0g	7g	1g	0mg	3mg

Exchanges:

1½ Fat

Italian Dressing

This dressing is sure to be requested often. Vary the spices to suit your own taste.

1/2 cup (120 ml) olive oil
2 tablespoons cider vinegar
2 tablespoons lemon juice
1 garlic clove, minced
1 green onion, chopped
1/2 teaspoon dried leaf oregano
1/2 teaspoon dry mustard
2 tablespoons no-salt-added tomato juice

Combine all ingredients in a jar or container with a tight-fitting lid. Shake and let stand 1 hour before using. Shake vigorously before using. Makes about 1 cup (250 ml).

Each tablespoon contains:

Cal.	Cal. from Fat	Protein	Carb.	Total Fiber	Total Fat	Sat. Fat	Chol.	Sodium
62	61	0g	0g	0g	7g	1g	0mg	2mg

Exchanges:

1 1/2 Fat

Russian Dressing

For serving with fish, omit the chili sauce and you have Thousand Island dressing.

1/3 cup (85 g) nonfat mayonnaise
1/3 cup (85 g) plain nonfat yogurt
3 tablespoons chili sauce or low-sodium catsup
1 tablespoon minced green bell pepper
1 teaspoon minced fresh chives
1 teaspoon minced pimiento
2 tablespoons sweet pickle relish

In a small bowl, combine mayonnaise, yogurt and chile sauce or catsup. Stir in remaining ingredients. Refrigerate in a container with a tight-fitting lid. Makes about 1 cup (230 g).

Each tablespoon contains:

Cal.	Cal. from Fat	Protein	Carb.	Total Fiber	Total Fat	Sat. Fat	Chol.	Sodium
10	0	0g	2g	0g	0g	0g	0mg	53mg

Exchanges:

Free

Yogurt-Cucumber Dressing

Make this early in the day and let the flavors develop.

1 cucumber, peeled, seeded and shredded
1/2 cup (115 g) plain nonfat yogurt
2 tablespoons pine nuts
2 tablespoons chopped capers
1 tablespoon lemon juice
1/2 teaspoon garlic powder
1 tablespoon chopped fresh parsley

In a small bowl, combine shredded cucumber with remaining ingredients. Cover and chill before serving. Makes about 1¼ cups (280 g).

Each tablespoon contains:

Cal.	Cal. from Fat	Protein	Carb.	Total Fiber	Total Fat	Sat. Fat	Chol.	Sodium
15	8	1g	1g	0g	1g	0g	0mg	32mg

Exchanges:

Free

Green Chile Mayonnaise

Wake up the flavor of mayonnaise. Use this as a topping on broiled fish or chicken or as a sandwich spread.

1/2 cup (115 g) nonfat mayonnaise
2 green onions, chopped
3 whole green chiles, seeded
1/4 teaspoon dried leaf oregano
1 teaspoon lemon juice

Combine all ingredients in a food processor or blender. Process until thoroughly blended. Refrigerate in a container with a tight-fitting lid. Makes about 1 cup (230 g).

Each tablespoon contains:

Cal.	Cal. from Fat	Protein	Carb.	Total Fiber	Total Fat	Sat. Fat	Chol.	Sodium
9	0	0g	2g	0g	0g	0g	0mg	54mg

Exchanges:

Free

Cinnamon Applesauce

Rome Beauty and Gravenstein apples are good choices for this recipe.

6 large apples, peeled, cored and coarsely chopped
1/3 cup (80 ml) water or apple juice
1/4 teaspoon ground cinnamon
1/8 teaspoon ground nutmeg

Combine ingredients in a 3-quart (3-liter) nonstick saucepan. Bring to a boil. Cover and simmer 5 to 10 minutes or until apples are tender. For a smoother texture, purée in a food processor or blender. Cover and refrigerate until cool. Makes about 4 cups (900 g).

1/4 cup contains:

Cal.	Cal. from Fat	Protein	Carb.	Total Fiber	Total Fat	Sat. Fat	Chol.	Sodium
47	3	0g	12g	2g	0g	0g	0mg	0mg

Exchanges:

1 Fruit

Tomato-Yogurt Sauce

Although the taste will be slightly different, you can substitute drained canned tomatoes for fresh.

2 large tomatoes, peeled, seeded and chopped
1/2 teaspoon Worcestershire sauce
1/2 teaspoon reduced-sodium soy sauce
1/2 cup (115 g) plain nonfat yogurt
3 tablespoons chopped fresh parsley
1 tablespoon chopped fresh chives

In a small bowl, combine all ingredients. Cover and refrigerate at least 1 hour to let flavors blend. Stir well before using. Makes about 1 cup (230 g).

Each tablespoon contains:

Cal.	Cal. from Fat	Protein	Carb.	Total Fiber	Total Fat	Sat. Fat	Chol.	Sodium
10	1	1g	2g	0g	0g	0g	0mg	16mg

Exchanges:

Free

Cantaloupe Salsa

A great accompaniment for grilled fish or poultry. You'll be amazed at how well these flavors complement one another.

1 cup (230 g) cubed cantaloupe
1 tablespoon chopped fresh parsley
2 tablespoons chopped sweet red onion
1 roasted mild green chile, peeled, seeded and chopped
2 tablespoons chopped fresh cilantro

In a small bowl, combine all ingredients. Cover and refrigerate at least 20 minutes before serving. Makes about 1½ cups (340 g).

Each tablespoon contains:

Cal.	Cal. from Fat	Protein	Carb.	Total Fiber	Total Fat	Sat. Fat	Chol.	Sodium
3	0	0g	1g	0g	0g	0g	0mg	1mg

Exchanges:

Free

Papaya-Pineapple Salsa

Serve this tropical medley with barbecued pork or fish.

1 fresh papaya, peeled, seeded and diced
1 (8-ounce/230-g) can crushed unsweetened pineapple
   with juice
1 roasted green chile, peeled and chopped, or 1 jalapeño chile,
seeded and finely chopped
2 tablespoons minced red onion
1 teaspoon grated orange zest
1/4 teaspoon grated fresh ginger

In a small bowl, combine all ingredients. Refrigerate in a container with a tight-fitting lid. Makes about 2 cups (450 g).

Each tablespoon contains:

Cal.	Cal. from Fat	Protein	Carb.	Total Fiber	Total Fat	Sat. Fat	Chol.	Sodium
9	0	0g	2g	0g	0g	0g	0mg	0mg

Exchanges:

Free

Tomato Salsa

Found on dining tables throughout Mexico, this versatile topping is good with chicken, fish or even eggs. And it makes a great dip.

1/4 cup (30 g) chopped onion
2/3 cup (140 g) chopped, peeled roasted green chile
1/4 to 1/2 teaspoon chili powder
1 (8-ounce/230-g) can low-sodium tomato sauce
4 tomatoes, peeled, seeded and chopped
1 tablespoon chopped fresh cilantro or parsley

Combine all ingredients in a small container. Cover and refrigerate. Let flavors develop 2 to 3 hours before using. Makes about 2 cups (450 g).

Each tablespoon contains:

Cal.	Cal. from Fat	Protein	Carb.	Total Fiber	Total Fat	Sat. Fat	Chol.	Sodium
6	0	0g	1g	0g	0g	0g	0mg	2mg

Exchanges:

Free

Rice, Beans & Pasta

These days we keep hearing that we should eat more grains. After all, grains provide many of the vitamins, minerals, protein and fiber we need to maintain a balanced diet. You can easily work grains into your diet with just a little thought. Try the recipes for Golden Indian Rice, Chile Cheese Grits and Curried Barley Casserole in this chapter. For a change, try some of the less familiar grains, such as millet and quinoa, which have been eaten for centuries by people in other countries.

Beans are another great source of fiber and other important nutrients and may even lower blood cholesterol. Before preparing dried beans, rinse them in water and remove any debris or broken beans. Presoak the beans to shorten their cooking time. There are two basic methods: long and short. In the first, place the beans in a large bowl or pan that will accommodate at least double the amount of beans. Pour in water to cover the beans by 2 to 3 inches and soak 8 hours. In the short soaking method, place the beans in a pot and cover with water; bring to a boil and cook 2 minutes in rapidly boiling water. Cover, remove from the heat, and let stand about 1 hour. Drain off the water and replace with fresh water. Proceed to cook. When using canned beans, rinse with water and drain to reduce the sodium content.

Pasta is climbing to the top of our preferred-foods list. We're told explorer Marco Polo brought pasta from China to Italy. I, for one, will always be grateful! Pasta is versatile as well as nutritious and combines easily with other foods. It's delicious served hot or cold. Pasta made from semolina is still the most popular type. However, for variety, try other flavors, such as spinach, beet, carrot, tomato and whole wheat.

Making your own pasta is easy, especially with the wonderful pasta machines that roll and cut the dough for you. Fresh pasta, unlike dried, cooks very quickly. Be careful to avoid overcooking it.

Brown Rice & Fruit

Both dried and fresh fruits combine nicely with the nutty flavor of brown rice.

> **2 cups cooked brown rice (3/4 cup/100 g uncooked)**
> **2 tablespoons almonds, toasted**
> **4 dried figs, chopped**
> **1 celery stalk, chopped**
> **1 cup (170 g) seedless red grapes**
> **1/2 cup (115 g) orange low-fat yogurt**
> **1/4 cup (60 ml) orange juice**
> **1 orange, peeled and segmented**
> **1 tablespoon chopped fresh mint (optional)**

In a large bowl, toss together rice, almonds, figs, celery and grapes. In a cup, stir together yogurt and orange juice. Pour over rice mixture and stir to combine. Garnish with orange segments and fresh mint if desired. Cover and refrigerate until chilled. Makes 6 servings.

Each serving contains:

Cal.	Cal. from Fat	Protein	Carb.	Total Fiber	Total Fat	Sat. Fat	Chol.	Sodium
160	23	3g	33g	4g	3g	0g	1mg	18mg

Exchanges:

1 Bread/Starch, 1 Fruit, 1/2 Fat

Golden Indian Rice

Turmeric provides the beautiful color, walnuts the crunch, and raisins a touch of sweetness.

1 cup (250 ml) low-sodium chicken broth
1 cup (250 ml) water
1 cup (140 g) uncooked long-grain white rice
3/4 teaspoon turmeric
2 green onions, chopped
1/4 cup (30 g) chopped walnuts
1/4 cup (30 g) golden raisins

In a 2-quart (2-liter) nonstick skillet, bring broth and water to a boil. Stir in rice and turmeric. Cover and reduce heat to a simmer. Cook about 20 minutes or until rice is tender. Stir in green onions, walnuts and raisins. Gently toss with a fork to combine. Serve hot or cold. Makes 6 servings.

Each serving contains:

Cal.	Cal. from Fat	Protein	Carb.	Total Fiber	Total Fat	Sat. Fat	Chol.	Sodium
173	31	4g	32g	1g	3g	0g	1mg	23mg

Exchanges:

1 1/2 Bread/Starch, 1/2 Very Lean Meat/Protein, 1/2 Fruit, 1/2 Fat

Mexican Rice

This side dish teams well with most beef or chicken dishes.

1 cup (140 g) uncooked long-grain white rice
3/4 cup (85 g) chopped green bell pepper
1 cup (115 g) chopped onion
1/4 cup (30 g) diced celery
2 tablespoons chopped roasted mild green chile
1 garlic clove, minced
2 tomatoes, peeled and chopped
1/4 cup (30 g) frozen green peas
1 cup (250 ml) low-sodium chicken broth
1 cup (250 ml) water
1/2 teaspoon black pepper
1/2 teaspoon dried leaf oregano
1/2 teaspoon chili powder

Spray a large nonstick skillet with olive oil cooking spray; heat over medium heat. Add rice and sauté briefly; do not brown. Remove rice to a bowl. In same skillet, sauté bell pepper, onion, celery, green chile and garlic until onion is golden brown. Add tomatoes and peas. Return rice to skillet. Add broth and water to rice along with black pepper, oregano and chili powder. Cover, reduce heat to low, and simmer 20 to 25 minutes or until broth is absorbed. Fluff rice with a fork before serving. Makes 4 servings.

Each serving contains:

Cal.	Cal. from Fat	Protein	Carb.	Total Fiber	Total Fat	Sat. Fat	Chol.	Sodium
153	7	4g	33g	3g	1g	0g	1mg	70mg

Exchanges:

1½ Bread/Starch, 1½ Vegetable

Pilaf with Currants

Almonds and currants add extra texture to a traditional side dish.

2 teaspoons olive oil
1 onion, chopped
3 tablespoons dried currants or chopped raisins
3 tablespoons chopped blanched almonds
1/2 red bell pepper, seeded and chopped
1 cup (140 g) uncooked long-grain white rice
1/2 cup (70 g) broken vermicelli (1-inch/2.5 cm pieces)
1 cup (250 ml) water

Heat oil in a medium nonstick skillet; sauté onion. Add remaining ingredients. Bring to a boil; reduce heat. Cover and cook about 20 minutes or until rice is tender and liquid is absorbed. Fluff pilaf with a fork before serving. Makes 6 servings.

Variation

Pilaf Casserole: Add 1/2 cup cooked, chopped carrots and 1 cup cooked chopped chicken with other ingredients after sautéing onion.

Each serving contains:

Cal.	Cal. from Fat	Protein	Carb.	Total Fiber	Total Fat	Sat. Fat	Chol.	Sodium
197	41	5g	34g	2g	5g	1g	1mg	23mg

Exchanges:

2 Bread/Starch, 1/2 Vegetable, 1 Fat

Barbecued Beans

Serve with Cabbage and Carrot Slaw, page 63, and cornbread for a well-balanced meal.

2 bacon strips, cubed
1 onion, chopped
2 cups (450 g) cooked small white beans
3/4 cup (180 ml) water
1/2 cup (120 ml) brewed coffee
1/4 cup (60 ml) lemon juice or vinegar
1/4 cup (55 g) low-sodium tomato paste
1 1/2 teaspoons dry mustard
1 teaspoon unsweetened cocoa powder
1/2 teaspoon paprika
1/2 teaspoon chili powder

Spray a small nonstick skillet with vegetable cooking spray. Sauté bacon and onion. Remove to a 5 1/2-quart (5.5-liter) nonstick Dutch oven or heavy pot and add remaining ingredients. Stir to combine. Cover and simmer about 30 minutes. Makes 8 servings.

Each serving contains:

Cal.	Cal. from Fat	Protein	Carb.	Total Fiber	Total Fat	Sat. Fat	Chol.	Sodium
223	28	13g	37g	14g	3g	1g	4mg	152mg

Exchanges:

2 1/2 Bread/Starch, 1/2 Very Lean Meat/Protein, 1/2 Fat

Dried Lima Bean Casserole

Serve this unusual bean dish with chicken or beef.

4 cups (900 g) cooked dried lima beans, drained
1 onion, sliced
1 cup (250 ml) low-sodium chicken broth
3/4 cup (180 ml) dry white wine
1/2 teaspoon red pepper flakes
1 tablespoon chopped fresh cilantro
2 tablespoons grated lemon zest
1/2 teaspoon paprika
Salt and black pepper to taste

Combine all ingredients in a 5½-quart (5.5-liter) nonstick Dutch oven; bring to a boil. Cover, reduce heat, and simmer 30 minutes, stirring occasionally. Uncover and cook 15 minutes longer. Makes 6 servings.

Each serving contains:

Cal.	Cal. from Fat	Protein	Carb.	Total Fiber	Total Fat	Sat. Fat	Chol.	Sodium
197	5	12g	32g	8g	1g	0g	0mg	19mg

Exchanges:

2 Bread/Starch, 1 Very Lean Meat/Protein

Curried Barley Casserole

The fragrant spices in this barley dish will help you cultivate a taste for Indian flavors.

2 teaspoons olive oil
2 celery stalks, sliced
1 onion, chopped
1/2 cup (45 g) sliced mushrooms
1 cup (130 g) pearl barley
1 cup (250 ml) low-sodium chicken broth
1 cup (250 ml) water
1/4 cup (60 ml) dry white wine
2 teaspoons curry powder
1/2 teaspoon ground cumin
2 tablespoons chopped fresh parsley
1 tomato, seeded and chopped

Heat oil in a 5 1/2-quart (5.5-liter) nonstick Dutch oven. Add celery, onion, mushrooms and barley. Stir to coat. Add broth, water, wine, curry powder and cumin. Cover and cook about 45 minutes. Uncover; stir in parsley and tomato; cover and cook 7 to 10 minutes. Makes 8 servings.

Each serving contains:

Cal.	Cal. from Fat	Protein	Carb.	Total Fiber	Total Fat	Sat. Fat	Chol.	Sodium
120	16	3g	22g	5g	2g	0g	0mg	28mg

Exchanges:

1 1/2 Bread/Starch, 1/2 Fat

Fettuccine with Herbs & Walnuts

Serve as a side dish with steak or chicken.

8 ounces (230 g) fettuccine
1 tablespoon olive oil
4 tablespoons minced fresh parsley
2 teaspoons dried leaf oregano
2 teaspoons dried leaf basil
1 teaspoon dried leaf rosemary
2 garlic cloves, minced
3 tablespoons chopped walnuts, toasted
2 tablespoons grated low-sodium Parmesan cheese

Cook fettuccine according to package directions. Drain, cover, and set aside. In a small skillet, cook oil, parsley, oregano, basil, rosemary and garlic over low heat about 1 minute. Remove from heat; set aside. In a large serving dish, combine warm fettuccine, herb mixture, walnuts and Parmesan. Toss gently to combine. Serve at once. Makes 4 servings.

Each serving contains:

Cal.	Cal. from Fat	Protein	Carb.	Total Fiber	Total Fat	Sat. Fat	Chol.	Sodium
295	83	10g	45g	3g	9g	2g	2mg	14mg

Exchanges:

3 Bread/Starch, 1/2 Lean Meat/Protein, 1½ Fat

Italian Sausage Spaghetti

This recipe proves it isn't necessary to spend hours making a wonderful sauce.

1/4 pound (115 g) sweet Italian sausage
1/4 onion, chopped
1/2 green bell pepper, seeded and chopped
3 tomatoes, chopped
1 1/2 teaspoons dried Italian seasoning
1 (8-ounce/230-g) can low-sodium tomato sauce
1/4 cup (60 ml) water
12 ounces (340 g) spaghetti, cooked
Chopped fresh parsley

Slit open sausage and remove casing; crumble or slice. In a large nonstick skillet, brown sausage; drain excess fat. Add onion and sauté. Add bell pepper, tomatoes, Italian seasoning, tomato sauce and water. Cover and cook about 20 minutes. Serve over spaghetti. Sprinkle with chopped parsley. Makes 6 servings.

Each serving contains:

Cal.	Cal. from Fat	Protein	Carb.	Total Fiber	Total Fat	Sat. Fat	Chol.	Sodium
174	59	7g	23g	2g	7g	2g	14mg	154mg

Exchanges:

1 Bread/Starch, 1/2 Lean Meat/Protein, 1 1/2 Vegetable, 1 Fat

Macaroni-Olive Frittata

Turn that bit of extra pasta into a delightful entrée.

3 eggs or 1 cup (250 ml) egg substitute
1 tablespoon cornstarch
1 tablespoon capers
6 or 7 pitted ripe black olives, sliced
1 tablespoon chopped fresh parsley
1 tablespoon olive oil
1 tablespoon butter
1/4 medium onion, chopped
1/2 cup (55 g) chopped red bell pepper
1 cup (2 ounces/57 g) uncooked macaroni or
    other small pasta, cooked
2 tomatoes, seeded and chopped
Chopped fresh basil

Preheat broiler. In a bowl, beat eggs or egg substitute and cornstarch. Stir in capers, olives and parsley; set aside. In a medium nonstick skillet with a flameproof handle, heat oil and butter over medium heat. Add onion and bell pepper; sauté until softened. Add macaroni and stir together until heated. Remove from heat. Pour egg mixture evenly over all. Reduce heat to low, cover, and cook 5 to 7 minutes. Remove cover and place skillet under broiler for 5 minutes or until top is firm and lightly browned. Loosen edges and cut into wedges. Top each wedge with tomatoes and basil. Makes 6 servings.

Each serving contains:

Cal.	Cal. from Fat	Protein	Carb.	Total Fiber	Total Fat	Sat. Fat	Chol.	Sodium
131	67	5g	12g	1g	7g	2g	111mg	117mg

Exchanges:

1/2 Bread/Starch, 1/2 Lean Meat/Protein, 1/2 Vegetable, 1 Fat

Penne Primavera

Serve warm or chilled. Dinner is ready in 30 minutes.

1 (10-ounce/280-g) package frozen broccoli spears,
     thawed and sliced
1/4 cup (30 g) frozen green peas
1 zucchini, halved lengthwise and sliced
1 yellow bell pepper, seeded and sliced
2 garlic cloves, minced
1/4 cup (60 ml) dry red wine
3 tablespoons fresh parsley leaves
1 tablespoon dried leaf basil
1 teaspoon dried leaf oregano
1 (16-ounce/450-g) package penne pasta
2 tomatoes, chopped
Red pepper flakes (optional)

Spray a medium nonstick skillet with olive oil cooking spray.
Add broccoli, peas, zucchini, bell pepper, garlic and wine;
cook 5 to 7 minutes. Set aside. Combine parsley, basil and
oregano in a blender or food processor. Blend until parsley is
fine and moist. Cook pasta according to package directions.
Add parsley mixture and tomatoes and toss. Add sautéed
vegetables and toss. Sprinkle with red pepper flakes if desired.
Serve warm or chilled. Makes 8 servings.

Each serving contains:

Cal.	Cal. from Fat	Protein	Carb.	Total Fiber	Total Fat	Sat. Fat	Chol.	Sodium
241	13	7g	52g	9g	1g	0g	0mg	21mg

Exchanges:

3 Bread/Starch, 1 Vegetable

Pasta with Mediterranean Vegetables

Turn the bounty of the garden into a light meal.

1 tablespoon olive oil
1 onion, sliced
2 garlic cloves, minced
1 fennel bulb, trimmed and thinly sliced
1/2 green bell pepper, seeded and sliced
1/2 red bell pepper, seeded and sliced
1/2 yellow bell pepper, seeded and sliced
1 cup (85 g) sliced mushrooms
2 tomatoes, chopped
3/4 cup (180 ml) no-salt-added tomato juice
1 tablespoon chopped fresh parsley
1/2 teaspoon dried leaf thyme
1/2 teaspoon dried leaf basil
12 ounces (340 g) macaroni or other pasta, cooked
2 tablespoons grated low-sodium Parmesan cheese

In a 5 1/2-quart (5.5-liter) nonstick Dutch oven, heat oil. Sauté onion and garlic. Add remaining ingredients except pasta and Parmesan. Stir and cook over medium heat until vegetables are tender. Serve over cooked pasta. Sprinkle each serving with Parmesan. Makes 6 servings.

Each serving contains:

Cal.	Cal. from Fat	Protein	Carb.	Total Fiber	Total Fat	Sat. Fat	Chol.	Sodium
152	35	6g	25g	4g	4g	1g	20mg	48mg

Exchanges:

1 Bread/Starch, 2 Vegetable, 1 Fat

Zucchini & Fettuccine in Tomato Sauce

Tender young zucchini add extra flavor to this vegetarian entrée.

1 tablespoon olive oil
1/2 large onion, chopped
2 large garlic cloves, minced
4 tablespoons chopped fresh parsley
1 teaspoon dried leaf basil
1/4 teaspoon dried leaf oregano
1 (28-ounce/790-g) can unsalted tomatoes with juice
1/4 cup (60 ml) dry red wine
1/4 cup (55 g) low-sodium tomato paste
1/2 cup (120 ml) water
8 ounces (230 g) fettuccine
1 pound (450 g) zucchini, sliced
3 tablespoons grated low-sodium Parmesan cheese

In a large sauté pan, heat oil over medium heat; add onion, garlic, parsley, basil and oregano; sauté 2 to 3 minutes. Add tomatoes and juice, wine, tomato paste and water. Cover, reduce heat to low, and simmer 15 to 20 minutes. Meanwhile, cook pasta according to package directions, omitting salt. Add zucchini to tomato sauce, cover, and simmer 10 to 15 minutes or until zucchini is tender. In a large bowl, combine tomato sauce and pasta. Sprinkle with Parmesan. Makes 6 servings.

Each serving contains:

Cal.	Cal. from Fat	Protein	Carb.	Total Fiber	Total Fat	Sat. Fat	Chol.	Sodium
230	39	7g	42g	7g	4g	1g	2mg	31mg

Exchanges:

2 Bread/Starch, 2 Vegetable, 1 Fat

Chile-Cheese Grits

Grits take on a new character with south-of-the-border flavors.

2 cups (500 ml) low-sodium chicken broth
1 cup (250 ml) water
3/4 cup (115 g) quick-cooking hominy grits
1 (4-ounce/115-g) can diced green chiles, drained
1 tomato, peeled, seeded and chopped
1 tablespoon chopped fresh cilantro
1 tablespoon chopped fresh chives
1/4 cup (30 g) shredded reduced-fat, reduced-sodium
    Monterey Jack cheese

Heat broth and water to boiling in a 2-quart (2-liter) nonstick saucepan. Stirring constantly, slowly add grits. Cook and stir over medium heat until thickened. Stir in chiles, tomato, cilantro and chives. Stir in cheese. Makes 6 servings.

Each serving contains:

Cal.	Cal. from Fat	Protein	Carb.	Total Fiber	Total Fat	Sat. Fat	Chol.	Sodium
96	15	4g	17g	1g	2g	1g	5mg	298mg

Exchanges:

1 Bread/Starch, 1/2 Lean Meat/Protein, 1/2 Vegetable

Lentils & Tomatoes

Cinnamon and caraway add an unusual dimension to this hearty dish.

1 cup (170 g) dried lentils
1/2 onion, chopped
1/4 teaspoon caraway seeds
1 carrot, sliced
1/4 teaspoon black pepper
1 red bell pepper, seeded and sliced
1/2 teaspoon ground cinnamon
2 cups (250 ml) water
1 (16-ounce/450-g) can no-salt-added tomatoes

Rinse and sort lentils. In a 3-quart (3-liter) nonstick saucepan, combine all ingredients. Bring to a boil. Cover, reduce heat, and simmer about 30 minutes or until lentils are done. Makes 6 servings.

Each serving contains:

Cal.	Cal. from Fat	Protein	Carb.	Total Fiber	Total Fat	Sat. Fat	Chol.	Sodium
126	5	9g	24g	8g	1g	0g	0mg	121mg

Exchanges:

1 Bread/Starch, 1/2 Very Lean Meat/Protein, 1½ Vegetable

Vegetables

It is difficult to imagine what our meals would be like without vegetables. They provide nutrition, color, texture and flavor. Today, thanks to rapid shipping, we can enjoy fresh produce year-round from faraway places.

The government's new food pyramid recommends that we consume five or six servings of vegetables and fruits a day. An easy way to increase your consumption of vegetables is simply to take your favorite casserole or stir-fry recipe, reduce the meat by half, and double the vegetables. When planning a side dish, forget the usual peas and carrots and introduce your family to vegetables that may be less familiar. Try Brussels Sprouts in Mustard Sauce, Leeks with Tarragon Sauce or Baked Portobello Mushrooms.

One nice way to prepare all types of vegetables is to steam them. You don't need special equipment, although steamers are handy. Simply place vegetables of uniform size in a vegetable-steamer basket, a strainer or colander, or on a rack above a small amount of simmering water. Cover and cook until they reach the desired tenderness, adding more water if needed. The water may be seasoned with a tablespoon of lemon juice or wine or with a pinch of herbs. Once again, be inventive—my recipes are just a guide to get you started in creative cooking.

Serve steamed vegetables plain or adorned with seasonings, yogurt or dressing. I like to serve at least two vegetables of contrasting color and texture with dinner. Think of the dinner plate as a painting: Vegetables supply the accents that complete the picture; they please the eye as well as the palate.

Asparagus Stir-Fry

Enjoy the short season of fresh asparagus with this colorful stir-fried side dish.

1 pound (450 g) fresh asparagus
2 teaspoons vegetable oil
1 garlic clove, minced
1 tablespoon minced fresh ginger
1/2 teaspoon Chinese five-spice powder
2 green onions, sliced
1/2 red bell pepper, seeded and sliced
1/4 cup (60 ml) water
1/2 teaspoon sesame oil (optional)

Trim tough asparagus ends and cut diagonally into 1 1/2-inch (4-cm) pieces. In a wok or large skillet, heat oil. Add garlic and ginger; cook, stirring, about 30 seconds. Add five-spice powder, green onions, bell pepper, asparagus and water. Stir-fry until vegetables are tender-crisp, about 3 minutes. If desired, add sesame oil to edge of pan and toss vegetables to mix. Makes 4 servings.

Each serving contains:

Cal.	Cal. from Fat	Protein	Carb.	Total Fiber	Total Fat	Sat. Fat	Chol.	Sodium
54	23	4g	6g	2g	3g	0g	0mg	5mg

Exchanges:

1 1/2 Vegetable, 1/2 Fat

Broccoli with Pine Nuts

A powerhouse of nutrients, broccoli takes well to "dressing up" for a change of pace.

1 pound (450 g) broccoli crowns
2 bacon strips, chopped
2 tablespoons pine nuts
1 tablespoon lime juice

Cook broccoli in a steamer 5 to 7 minutes or until tender. Place in a serving bowl and cover. In a small nonstick skillet, cook bacon, stirring, until crisp. Remove from heat and add pine nuts and lime juice. Stir to combine and pour over broccoli. Serve at once. Makes 6 servings.

Each serving contains:

Cal.	Cal. from Fat	Protein	Carb.	Total Fiber	Total Fat	Sat. Fat	Chol.	Sodium
88	57	5g	5g	1g	6g	2g	5mg	126mg

Exchanges:

1/2 Lean Meat/Protein, 1 Vegetable, 1 Fat

Brussels Sprouts in Mustard Sauce

Mild mustard sauce is a traditional pairing with Brussels sprouts.

**1 (10-ounce/280-g) package frozen or 3/4 pound (340 g)
   fresh Brussels sprouts**
1 1/2 cups (375 ml) low-sodium chicken broth
1 teaspoon canola oil
2 tablespoons chopped green onion
1 teaspoon dry mustard
1/2 teaspoon black pepper
1 tablespoon cornstarch
1/2 cup (120 ml) evaporated skimmed milk

Cook Brussels sprouts in 1/2 cup (120 ml) broth in a 2-quart (2-liter) nonstick saucepan; cover and set aside. Spray a small nonstick skillet with vegetable cooking spray. Add oil and sauté green onion. Remove from heat and slowly add remaining 1 cup (250 ml) broth. Stir in mustard and pepper. Return to heat. Dissolve cornstarch in evaporated milk. Pour into mixture. Stirring constantly, cook until sauce is smooth and thickened, about 5 minutes. Pour mustard sauce over cooked Brussels sprouts and stir to coat. Serve at once. Makes 4 servings.

Each serving contains:

Cal.	Cal. from Fat	Protein	Carb.	Total Fiber	Total Fat	Sat. Fat	Chol.	Sodium
79	13	6g	12g	3g	1g	0g	3mg	94mg

Exchanges:

1/2 Bread/Starch, 1 Vegetable, 1/2 Skim Milk

Eggplant Casserole

Orange and tomato add a piquant flavor to otherwise bland eggplant.

1 pound (450 g) eggplant, cut into 8 slices
1/2 teaspoon salt
2 tablespoons olive oil
2 green onions, chopped
2 garlic cloves, minced
4 teaspoons cornstarch
1/2 cup (120 ml) orange juice
1/2 cup (120 ml) low-sodium chicken broth
1/2 cup (120 ml) evaporated skimmed milk
1/2 teaspoon poultry seasoning
1/4 teaspoon black pepper
1 teaspoon grated orange zest
1 cup (85 g) sliced mushrooms
1 cup (170 g) chopped cooked chicken breast
2 cups cooked white rice (3/4 cup/100 g uncooked)
2 tomatoes

Sprinkle eggplant slices with salt; set aside 30 minutes. Pat with paper towels to remove excess moisture. Brush slices with 1 tablespoon oil and brown on both sides in a large nonstick skillet. In a medium nonstick skillet, heat remaining tablespoon oil and sauté green onions and garlic. Dissolve cornstarch in orange juice and broth; stir into onion and garlic. Add evaporated milk, poultry seasoning, pepper and orange zest. When mixture has thickened, add mushrooms and chicken. Stir to combine. Spoon rice into a 5½-quart (5.5-liter) Dutch oven. Place eggplant slices in one layer over rice. Cut each tomato in 4 slices and place on top of eggplant. Pour mushroom-chicken sauce over all. Cover and cook over low heat about 20 minutes. Makes 8 servings.

Each serving contains:

Cal.	Cal. from Fat	Protein	Carb.	Total Fiber	Total Fat	Sat. Fat	Chol.	Sodium
162	41	9g	22g	2g	5g	1g	15mg	184mg

Exchanges:

1 Bread/Starch, 1 Very Lean Meat/Protein, 1 Vegetable, 1 Fat

Spicy Green Beans

Cauliflower and carrots may be treated in the same manner.

**2 pounds (900 g) fresh or 2 (10-ounce/280-g) packages
    frozen green beans**
1 cup (115 g) chopped jícama or water chestnuts
2 tablespoons chopped fresh parsley
3 tablespoons chopped pimiento-stuffed olives
1/2 cup (120 ml) Italian Dressing (page 83)

Trim ends of fresh green beans. Cook in water to cover in a
3-quart (3-liter) nonstick saucepan 10 to 12 minutes or until
tender-crisp; drain. If using frozen beans, cook according to
package directions; drain. Combine beans, jícama or water
chestnuts, parsley and olives in a shallow bowl. Pour dressing
over bean mixture. Cover and refrigerate at least 2 hours.
Stir mixture twice while chilling it. Makes 6 servings.

Each serving contains:

Cal.	Cal. from Fat	Protein	Carb.	Total Fiber	Total Fat	Sat. Fat	Chol.	Sodium
60	7	3g	13g	6g	1g	0g	0mg	108mg

Exchanges:

2 1/2 Vegetable

Leeks with Tarragon Sauce

Members of the onion family, such as leeks, are typically served in a white sauce, but no one will guess this one is low in fat.

4 leeks
1 cup (250 ml) low-sodium chicken broth
1/2 cup (120 ml) water
1 teaspoon dried leaf tarragon
1/4 cup (60 ml) white vermouth or lemon juice
1/2 cup (55 g) chopped red bell pepper
2 tablespoons cornstarch
1/4 cup (60 ml) fat-free milk
1 tablespoon chopped fresh chives
Black pepper to taste

Trim dark green portion and roots from leeks. Cut in half lengthwise; thoroughly rinse to remove dirt. In a large nonstick skillet, heat broth and water; add leeks, cover, and simmer 7 to 10 minutes or until tender. Remove leeks to a serving dish; cover and keep warm. Add tarragon, vermouth or lemon juice and bell pepper to broth. Dissolve cornstarch in milk. Stir into broth. Over medium heat, continue stirring until thickened. Add chives. Season to taste with black pepper. Pour sauce over leeks. Serve at once. Makes 4 servings.

Each serving contains:

Cal.	Cal. from Fat	Protein	Carb.	Total Fiber	Total Fat	Sat. Fat	Chol.	Sodium
112	7	3g	21g	2g	1g	0g	1mg	56mg

Exchanges:

1/2 Bread/Starch, 3 Vegetable

Baked Portobello Mushrooms

Serve these meaty mushrooms as a side dish for steak.

1 pound (450 g) portobello mushrooms, sliced
1 red onion, chopped
4 teaspoons chopped hazelnuts
1 to 2 tablespoons balsamic vinegar

Preheat oven to 400F (200C). Spray a shallow baking dish with olive oil cooking spray. Place mushrooms in dish in a single layer. Lightly spray with olive oil. Top mushrooms with onion and hazelnuts. Drizzle balsamic vinegar over all. Bake about 15 minutes. Makes 4 servings.

Each serving contains:

Cal.	Cal. from Fat	Protein	Carb.	Total Fiber	Total Fat	Sat. Fat	Chol.	Sodium
59	18	3g	9g	2g	2g	0g	0mg	7mg

Exchanges:

1½ Vegetable, 1/2 Fat

Sweet Potato Fritters

Fritters make a pretty side dish that departs from the ordinary.

1 (8-ounce/230-g) sweet potato, peeled and shredded
1 carrot, shredded
1 tablespoon minced onion
2 eggs or 1/2 cup (120 ml) egg substitute
1/4 cup (35 g) all-purpose flour
3 tablespoons orange juice
1 tablespoon grated orange zest
2 tablespoons chopped fresh parsley
1 to 2 tablespoons canola oil

In a medium bowl, thoroughly combine all ingredients except oil. In a large nonstick skillet, heat 1 tablespoon oil. For each fritter, carefully spoon about 2 tablespoons sweet potato mixture into pan. Press lightly to form fritters. When edges begin to brown, turn and lightly press again; cook other side. Place on paper towels, cover to keep warm, and continue to cook fritters, adding more oil as needed. Makes 10 fritters.

Each fritter contains:

Cal.	Cal. from Fat	Protein	Carb.	Total Fiber	Total Fat	Sat. Fat	Chol.	Sodium
81	35	2g	10g	1g	4g	1g	43mg	19mg

Exchanges:

1/2 Bread/Starch, 1/2 Vegetable, 1 Fat

Spinach-Rice Stuffed Peppers

For added color, use a mixture of orange, red and yellow bell peppers.

1 (10-ounce/280-g) package frozen chopped spinach, thawed
2 teaspoons olive oil
1 small onion, minced
1 garlic clove, minced
1/4 cup (30 g) corn kernels
1/4 teaspoon dried leaf basil
1/4 teaspoon dried leaf oregano
2 tablespoons raisins
1/2 cup (115 g) cooked brown rice
2 tablespoons no-salt-added tomato paste
1 egg white, slightly beaten
4 bell peppers, seeded and stemmed
2 teaspoons chopped pimiento
2 teaspoons chopped fresh parsley

Preheat oven to 375F (190C). Spray a 10 x 8-inch (25 x 20-cm) baking dish with olive oil cooking spray. Drain spinach, squeezing out as much liquid as possible. Set aside. In an small nonstick skillet, heat oil; sauté onion and garlic. In a large mixing bowl, combine spinach, corn, basil, oregano, raisins, rice, tomato paste and egg white. Fill peppers with mixture and top with pimiento and parsley. Place in prepared baking dish. Bake about 30 minutes. Makes 4 servings.

Each serving contains:

Cal.	Cal. from Fat	Protein	Carb.	Total Fiber	Total Fat	Sat. Fat	Chol.	Sodium
126	28	5g	22g	5g	3g	0g	0mg	79mg

Exchanges:

1/2 Bread/Starch, 2½ Vegetable, 1/2 Fat

Potato Sticks

Serve these wedges with Hamburgers Supreme, page 145, or baked chicken.

2 large baking potatoes, unpeeled
1 tablespoon olive oil
1 teaspoon anise seeds
1 teaspoon paprika
Black pepper to taste

Preheat oven to 425F (220C). Scrub potatoes and pat dry. Cut each into 8 wedges. Brush with oil and place in a baking dish. Sprinkle with anise seeds and paprika. Bake about 35 minutes or until potatoes are tender. Season with pepper. Makes 4 servings.

Each serving contains:

Cal.	Cal. from Fat	Protein	Carb.	Total Fiber	Total Fat	Sat. Fat	Chol.	Sodium
106	32	2g	17g	1g	4g	0g	0mg	4mg

Exchanges:

1 Bread/Starch, 1 Fat

Garlic Baked Potatoes

Make ahead, cover and refrigerate until ready to reheat.

3 medium baking potatoes
1/4 cup (55 g) plain nonfat yogurt
1/2 cup (115 g) nonfat cottage cheese
1 tablespoon chopped fresh chives
1 tablespoon garlic paste
2 teaspoons chopped fresh parsley
4 tablespoons grated low-sodium Parmesan cheese
Paprika

Preheat oven to 425F (220C) and bake potatoes about
1 hour. Remove from oven and lower oven temperature to
375F (190C). Slice potatoes in half lengthwise and carefully
scoop out pulp, leaving shells intact. Place shells on a baking
sheet. In a large mixing bowl, mash potato pulp with yogurt,
cottage cheese, chives, garlic paste, parsley and 2 tablespoons
Parmesan. Fill potato shells, mounding mixture. Sprinkle with
remaining cheese and paprika. Bake 15 to 20 minutes or until
heated through. Makes 6 servings.

Each serving contains:

Cal.	Cal. from Fat	Protein	Carb.	Total Fiber	Total Fat	Sat. Fat	Chol.	Sodium
95	19	4g	16g	1g	2g	1g	4mg	28mg

Exchanges:

1 Bread/Starch, 1/2 Lean Meat/Protein

Squash-Cheese Casserole

A colorful medley of vegetables, sure to please almost everyone.

2 crookneck squash, sliced
2 patty pan squash, sliced
2 tomatoes, sliced
1 (12-ounce/340-g) can cream-style corn
3 green onions, chopped
6 (2/3-ounce/20-g) slices low-fat American cheese
2 teaspoons chopped fresh tarragon or
   1/2 teaspoon dried leaf tarragon

Preheat oven to 350F (175C). Spray a 2-quart (2-liter) casserole with vegetable cooking spray. Combine squash, tomatoes, corn and green onions. Cover and bake 20 minutes. Place cheese slices in one layer over vegetables. Scatter tarragon on top of cheese. Bake, uncovered, 10 to 12 minutes. Makes 6 servings.

Each serving contains:

Cal.	Cal. from Fat	Protein	Carb.	Total Fiber	Total Fat	Sat. Fat	Chol.	Sodium
80	8	3g	18g	3g	1g	0g	1mg	55mg

Exchanges:

1 Bread/Starch, 1/2 Vegetable

Baked Mixed Vegetables

When preparing roast beef, add this dish to the oven during the last minutes of cooking the meat.

1 (16-ounce/450-g) package frozen mixed vegetables
1 cup (250 ml) low-sodium beef broth
1/2 teaspoon dried leaf basil
1/2 teaspoon dried leaf tarragon
2 teaspoons chopped fresh parsley

Preheat oven to 350F (175C). Combine all ingredients in a shallow baking dish. Bake, covered, about 20 minutes, stirring occasionally. Serve hot or cold. Makes 5 servings.

Each serving contains:

Cal.	Cal. from Fat	Protein	Carb.	Total Fiber	Total Fat	Sat. Fat	Chol.	Sodium
63	6	4g	13g	4g	1g	0g	0mg	51mg

Exchanges:

1 Bread/Starch

Dilled Vegetables

A colorful medley of favorite vegetables.

2 teaspoons olive oil
1/2 pound (230 g) pearl onions, peeled
1 pound (450 g) small new potatoes, cubed
4 carrots, sliced
1 cup (250 ml) low-sodium chicken broth
1 (10-ounce/280-g) package frozen broccoli spears, thawed
1 cup (114 g) frozen sugar snap pea pods
1/2 teaspoon dill weed
1/3 cup (85 g) plain nonfat yogurt

Heat oil in a 5½-quart (5.5-liter) nonstick Dutch oven. Sauté onions until lightly browned. Add potatoes, carrots and broth; heat to boiling. Reduce to a simmer, cover, and cook 30 to 45 minutes or until vegetables are tender. Add broccoli and pea pods; cook 5 minutes longer. Stir dill weed into yogurt. Spoon over cooked vegetables. Makes 6 servings.

Each serving contains:

Cal.	Cal. from Fat	Protein	Carb.	Total Fiber	Total Fat	Sat. Fat	Chol.	Sodium
129	19	6g	23g	5g	2g	0g	1mg	56mg

Exchanges:

1 Bread/Starch, 2 Vegetable, 1/2 Fat

Fish & Seafood

The bounty of the sea waits for you at your market. Although fresh seafood is preferable, it's not always available. Fortunately, frozen seafood can be a very satisfactory substitute. Modern processing at sea results in quick freezing, which helps preserve flavor and texture.

If you have a fishing enthusiast in the family, encourage him or her to bring home the catch. To freeze fish at home—a slower process than commercial freezing—place it in a shallow pan, fill with water, cover with foil, and freeze. After it is frozen solid, transfer the "fish-sicle" to a plastic freezer bag.

Try to include fish in your diet two or three times a week. It's low in calories and high in protein. And don't overlook the benefits of consuming the omega-3 fatty acids contained in oily fish, which have many benefits for your heart, including lowering cholesterol. Herring, mackerel, salmon, trout, and white tuna are some of the best sources of omega-3 fatty acids. However, these benefits can be lost when the fish is deep-fried or heavily sauced with butter or cream. The healthiest way to cook any fish is to bake, broil, grill, poach, stir-fry, or steam it. For best results, cook fish over high heat for a short time; overcooking both toughens and dries out fish.

Ease of preparation and short cooking time make fish or seafood an ideal choice on busy days. Enjoy Tuna & Pasta if you are in the mood for something cold. For a special occasion, choose Orange Roughy Packets or Oriental-Style Fillets. Tender Scallop Kabobs taste so good that no one will suspect they were prepared in minutes. If you love salmon, be sure to treat yourself to the Salmon with Curry Sauce.

Baked Sea Bass in Salsa

You decide how hot to make the salsa by selecting either the mild Anaheim chile or the hotter jalapeño.

1/4 onion, chopped
1 cup (230 g) chopped tomatoes
1 cup (230 g) chopped fresh tomatillos
1 Anaheim or jalapeño chile, seeded and chopped
1/2 teaspoon dried leaf oregano
1 pound (450 g) sea bass fillets

Preheat oven to 425F (220C). Spray a medium nonstick skillet with olive oil cooking spray. Add onion, tomatoes, and tomatillos. Sauté over medium-high heat 3 to 5 minutes. Add chile and oregano. Sauté 3 to 5 minutes longer. Rinse fillets and pat dry. Place fillets in a single layer in a baking pan. Spoon tomato mixture on top. Cover and cook about 10 minutes or until fish flakes. Serve at once. Makes 4 servings.

Each serving contains:

Cal.	Cal. from Fat	Protein	Carb.	Total Fiber	Total Fat	Sat. Fat	Chol.	Sodium
143	30	22g	6g	1g	3g	1g	96mg	87mg

Exchanges:

3 Lean Meat/Protein, 1 Vegetable, 1/2 Fat

Crisp Catfish Fillets

It may be hard to believe, but it is possible to have a crisp coating without frying.

1 pound (450 g) skinless catfish fillets
1/2 cup (120 ml) evaporated skimmed milk
1/3 cup (55 g) cornmeal
1/4 teaspoon cayenne pepper
1 teaspoon dried leaf thyme
1 teaspoon dried leaf oregano
1/4 teaspoon garlic powder

Preheat oven to 400F (200C). Lightly spray a baking dish with vegetable cooking spray. Rinse fillets and pat dry. Set aside. Pour evaporated milk into a shallow dish or pie plate. In another dish, combine cornmeal, cayenne, thyme, oregano, and garlic powder. Dip each fillet in milk, then in cornmeal mixture. Place in prepared baking dish. Bake 10 to 12 minutes or until golden brown and fish flakes. Makes 4 servings.

Each serving contains:

Cal.	Cal. from Fat	Protein	Carb.	Total Fiber	Total Fat	Sat. Fat	Chol.	Sodium
178	32	22g	13g	1g	4g	1g	67mg	86mg

Exchanges:

1/2 Bread/Starch, 3 Very Lean Meat/Protein, 1/2 Skim Milk, 1/2 Fat

Pasta with Clam & Tomato Sauce

Try this Sicilian favorite for your next pasta meal. Best of all, it's ready in less than 30 minutes.

2 teaspoons olive oil
1 garlic clove
1/4 onion, chopped
1/4 green bell pepper, chopped
2 teaspoons grated lemon zest
2 teaspoons chopped fresh parsley
1/2 teaspoon dried leaf oregano
1 large tomato, seeded and chopped
3 tablespoons lemon juice
1 (6-ounce/170-g) can clams
1/2 cup (70 g) frozen green peas
8 ounces (230 g) ziti, cooked
4 teaspoons grated low-sodium Parmesan cheese

In a medium nonstick skillet, heat oil. Add garlic, onion, and bell pepper and sauté about 3 minutes until softened, not browned. Stir in lemon zest, parsley, oregano, tomato, and lemon juice. Reduce heat; add clams with juice. Cover and simmer 15 minutes. Add peas and cook 5 minutes. Serve over cooked pasta and sprinkle with Parmesan cheese. Makes 4 servings.

Each serving contains:

Cal.	Cal. from Fat	Protein	Carb.	Total Fiber	Total Fat	Sat. Fat	Chol.	Sodium
142	32	5g	23g	3g	4g	1g	3mg	121mg

Exchanges:

1½ Bread/Starch, 1/2 Vegetable, 1 Fat

Broiled Cod

Scallops, sea bass, or shrimp can be substituted for cod.

1 (12-ounce/375-ml) can beer
1/4 teaspoon red pepper flakes
1/2 teaspoon dry mustard
1 tablespoon lime juice
2 green onions, chopped
1/4 teaspoon paprika
1/2 to 3/4 pound (230 to 340 g) cod fillets

In a baking dish, mix beer, red pepper flakes, mustard, lime juice, green onions, and paprika. Add cod; marinate 3 to 4 hours, covered and refrigerated. Preheat broiler to 450F (230C) or high. Spray broiler pan with vegetable cooking spray and arrange fillets in a single layer. Broil 7 to 10 minutes or until fish flakes. Turn at least once, brushing with more marinade if necessary. Serve at once. Makes 4 servings.

Each serving contains:

Cal.	Cal. from Fat	Protein	Carb.	Total Fiber	Total Fat	Sat. Fat	Chol.	Sodium
101	6	16g	3g	0g	1g	0g	37mg	52mg

Exchanges:

2 Very Lean Meat/Protein

Oriental-Style Fillets

Popular flavors from the Pacific Rim give fish an innovative twist.

1 pound (450 g) white fish fillets
1/4 cup (60 ml) reduced-sodium soy sauce
2 tablespoons lime juice
1 tablespoon grated lime zest
1 teaspoon canola oil
2 teaspoons grated fresh ginger
2 green onions, sliced
1 teaspoon toasted sesame seeds, for garnish

Arrange fish fillets in a baking dish. Combine soy sauce, lime juice, lime zest, oil, ginger, and green onions in a small mixing bowl. Pour over fish. Turn fillets to coat both sides. Cover and refrigerate at least 1 hour. Drain and reserve marinade. Preheat broiler; spray broiler pan with vegetable cooking spray and arrange fillets on broiler pan. Broil 3 to 4 minutes on each side or until fish flakes, brushing with marinade at least once. Sprinkle with sesame seeds. Makes 4 servings.

Each serving contains:

Cal.	Cal. from Fat	Protein	Carb.	Total Fiber	Total Fat	Sat. Fat	Chol.	Sodium
187	79	23g	5g	1g	8g	1g	70mg	594mg

Exchanges:

3 Very Lean Meat/Protein, 1/2 Vegetable, 1½ Fat

Curried Halibut Steaks

The steaks can be poached ahead of time and broiled just before serving.

1 quart (1 l) water
3 slices fresh ginger
2 slices lemon
1/4 cup (60 ml) dry vermouth
2 tablespoons chopped celery leaves
1 pound (450 g) halibut steaks, about 1 inch (2.5 cm) thick
1/3 cup (85 g) plain nonfat yogurt
3 tablespoons nonfat mayonnaise
1/2 teaspoon dill weed
2 teaspoons minced fresh chives
1/4 teaspoon black pepper
1 teaspoon curry powder
Lemon wedges

In a large saucepan or fish cooker, combine water, ginger, lemon slices, vermouth, and celery leaves. Bring to a simmer. Add halibut steaks; cover and simmer 4 minutes or until barely done. With slotted spoon or spatula, carefully lift fish out of water; place on a broiler pan. At this point, you can cover and refrigerate halibut until needed. Preheat broiler. In a small bowl, combine yogurt, mayonnaise, dill weed, chives, pepper, and curry powder. Spread over top of each steak. Broil 5 to 6 inches (13 to 15 cm) from heat source until bubbly and golden on top. Garnish with lemon wedges. Makes 4 servings.

Each serving contains:

Cal.	Cal. from Fat	Protein	Carb.	Total Fiber	Total Fat	Sat. Fat	Chol.	Sodium
167	24	25g	6g	0g	3g	0g	37mg	160mg

Exchanges:

3 1/2 Very Lean Meat/Protein, 1/2 Fat

Mahi Mahi with Tomatoes

Hawaiians introduced us to this delicious, meaty fish from the Pacific.

2 teaspoons olive oil
1 onion, chopped
2 garlic cloves, chopped
3 tomatoes, chopped
1 roasted green chile, peeled, seeded, and chopped
3 tablespoons chopped fresh parsley
1 pound (450 g) mahi mahi or cod, cut into 1-inch
     (2.5-cm) cubes
2 tablespoons sliced toasted almonds

In a medium nonstick skillet, heat oil. Add onion and garlic and sauté until softened, not browned, about 3 minutes. Add tomatoes, chile, and parsley. Cook together 3 to 4 minutes. Add fish cubes, cover, and cook 10 minutes. Sprinkle with almonds. Makes 4 servings.

Each serving contains:

Cal.	Cal. from Fat	Protein	Carb.	Total Fiber	Total Fat	Sat. Fat	Chol.	Sodium
175	47	23g	9g	2g	5g	1g	83mg	112mg

Exchanges:

3 Very Lean Meat/Protein, 1½ Vegetable, 1 Fat

Orange Roughy in Packets

Baking fish and vegetables together in parchment or foil gives succulent results. And there's no mess to clean up.

1 carrot, julienned
1/4 red bell pepper, sliced
6 whole Chinese snow pea pods
2 (6-ounce/170-g) orange roughy or cod fillets
2 tablespoons lime juice
Paprika
2 tablespoons capers
2 tablespoons chopped parsley

Preheat oven to 425F (220C). Precook carrot in 1/2 cup (120 ml) water in a small saucepan for 5 minutes. Drain and set aside. Cut parchment or foil into 2 pieces large enough to wrap each fillet. Place half of carrot, bell pepper, and pea pods in center of each piece. Place 1 fillet on top of vegetables. Pour lime juice over fillets and sprinkle with paprika. Top with capers and parsley. Fold parchment or foil edges together; roll and fold to seal. Place on a baking sheet and bake 8 to 10 minutes. To serve, place packet on serving dish, cut a slash in top, and tear open. Makes 2 servings.

Each serving contains:

Cal.	Cal. from Fat	Protein	Carb.	Total Fiber	Total Fat	Sat. Fat	Chol.	Sodium
173	19	31g	6g	2g	2g	0g	73mg	511mg

Exchanges:

4½ Very Lean Meat/Protein, 1 Vegetable

Salmon with Curry Sauce

Enjoy the delicate flavor of salmon topped with a mild curry sauce.

1 pound (450 g) salmon fillets
1 tablespoon canola oil
1 tablespoon chopped fresh chives
1 tablespoon curry powder
1 teaspoon dry mustard
1/4 cup (60 ml) dry white wine
2 tablespoons lemon juice
1 tablespoon dried currants
1 teaspoon cornstarch
3/4 cup (180 ml) evaporated skimmed milk

Preheat broiler. Spray broiler pan with vegetable cooking spray. Rinse fillets and pat dry. Lightly spray with vegetable cooking spray and broil about 10 minutes per inch of fish. In a nonstick skillet, heat oil. Stir in chives, curry powder, and mustard. Blend thoroughly. Remove from heat; stirring constantly, add wine and lemon juice. Return to heat and add currants. Dissolve cornstarch in evaporated milk; stir into curry mixture until blended. Remove broiled fish to serving dishes and top with curry sauce. Serve at once. Makes 4 servings.

Each serving contains:

Cal.	Cal. from Fat	Protein	Carb.	Total Fiber	Total Fat	Sat. Fat	Chol.	Sodium
254	98	26g	9g	1g	11g	1g	64mg	109mg

Exchanges:

3 Lean Meat/Protein, 1/2 Skim Milk, 1/2 Fat

Red Snapper with Vermouth

Red pepper and peas add color and interest to a wine sauce touched with the merest hint of cinnamon.

1 teaspoon olive oil
1 green onion, chopped
1/4 cup (30 g) sliced red bell pepper
1 garlic clove, minced
1/4 teaspoon ground cinnamon
3/4 cup (180 ml) dry vermouth
1/2 cup (70 g) frozen petite peas
1 pound (450 g) red snapper fillets

In a medium nonstick skillet, heat oil and sauté green onion, bell pepper, garlic, and cinnamon. Add vermouth and peas. Rinse fillets and pat dry. Place in pan. Spoon mixture over fillets. Cover and cook 5 minutes. Remove lid, spoon sauce over fish, and cook another 5 minutes. Serve with sauce. Makes 4 servings.

Each serving contains:

Cal.	Cal. from Fat	Protein	Carb.	Total Fiber	Total Fat	Sat. Fat	Chol.	Sodium
212	25	24g	9g	1g	3g	0g	42mg	98mg

Exchanges:

1/2 Bread/Starch, 3½ Very Lean Meat/Protein, 1/2 Fat

Scallop Kabobs

The delicate flavor of scallops is accented by the Italian Dressing.

1/2 cup (120 ml) Italian Dressing (page 83)
1 pound (450 g) scallops
1 small onion, quartered
1 red bell pepper, seeded and cubed
1 green bell pepper, seeded and cubed
12 small fresh mushrooms
2 cups cooked white rice (3/4 cup/100 g uncooked)

Pour Italian Dressing into a medium mixing bowl. Add scallops and onion, tossing to coat all pieces. Cover and refrigerate at least 2 hours. Preheat broiler. Thread scallops, onion, bell peppers, and mushrooms onto skewers. Broil, turning often, about 7 minutes. Serve with steamed rice. Makes 4 servings.

Each serving contains:

Cal.	Cal. from Fat	Protein	Carb.	Total Fiber	Total Fat	Sat. Fat	Chol.	Sodium
197	22	13g	31g	2g	2g	0g	18mg	237mg

Exchanges:

1 1/2 Bread/Starch, 1 1/2 Very Lean Meat/Protein, 1 1/2 Vegetable, 1/2 Fat

Shrimp & Cashew Stir-Fry

If snow peas are not available, substitute petit peas.

2 teaspoons rice wine or dry sherry
2 teaspoons reduced-sodium soy sauce
1 pound (450 g) fresh shrimp, shelled and deveined
1 tablespoon canola oil
2 teaspoons grated fresh ginger
1 green onion, including top, chopped
1 garlic clove, minced
1 (10-ounce/280-g) package frozen snow peas, thawed
1/4 cup (30 g) cashews
2 to 3 drops sesame oil
2 cups cooked white rice (3/4 cup/100 g uncooked)

In a medium bowl, combine rice wine or sherry and soy sauce. Add shrimp and toss to coat; set aside for 15 minutes. Heat oil in a large nonstick stir-fry pan. Add ginger, green onion, and garlic and sauté a few seconds. Drain shrimp and pat with paper towel. Add shrimp to pan and stir-fry, turning, 1 to 2 minutes. Add snow peas and cashews. Stir-fry 1 minute longer or until heated through. Remove from heat, drizzle with sesame oil, and toss to coat. Serve over rice. Makes 4 servings.

Each serving contains:

Cal.	Cal. from Fat	Protein	Carb.	Total Fiber	Total Fat	Sat. Fat	Chol.	Sodium
320	79	23g	36g	4g	9g	1g	161mg	291mg

Exchanges:

2 Bread/Starch, 2½ Very Lean Meat/Protein, 2 Fat

Baked Sole Fillets

Tomato, fennel and basil give mild sole Italian flair. Be careful not to overcook the fillets or they will dry out.

1 pound (450 g) sole fillets
1/2 teaspoon crushed fennel seeds
Black pepper to taste
1 garlic clove, minced
1½ cups (340 g) diced fresh tomato
2 green onions, diced
2 tablespoons chopped fresh basil or parsley

Preheat oven to 425F (220C). Spray a baking dish with olive oil cooking spray. Place fillets in a single layer in baking dish. Spray fillets with olive oil cooking spray. Combine fennel seeds, pepper, and garlic. Sprinkle over fish. Arrange tomatoes and green onions over fish. Sprinkle with basil or parsley. Cover with foil. Bake 10 to 15 minutes or until fish flakes. Makes 4 servings.

Each serving contains:

Cal.	Cal. from Fat	Protein	Carb.	Total Fiber	Total Fat	Sat. Fat	Chol.	Sodium
123	15	22g	4g	1g	2g	0g	54mg	100mg

Exchanges:

3 Very Lean Meat/Protein, 1 Vegetable

Sole Florentine

Mushrooms and pimiento brighten the creamed spinach filling.

2 teaspoons olive oil
1/2 onion, chopped
1 garlic clove, minced
2 tablespoons all-purpose flour
1 cup (250 ml) fat-free milk
1/4 cup (20 g) chopped mushrooms
2 tablespoons chopped pimiento
1/4 teaspoon ground nutmeg
1 (10-ounce/280-g) package frozen chopped spinach,
    thawed and drained
1 pound (450 g) sole fillets

Preheat oven to 425F (220C). In a 2-quart (2-liter) nonstick saucepan, heat oil. Add onion and garlic and sauté until soft but not browned, about 3 minutes. Stir in flour and milk. Cook, stirring, until thickened. Stir in mushrooms, pimiento, nutmeg, and spinach. Thoroughly combine. Lay fillets on a work surface and spread spinach mixture evenly over them. Roll up and secure with wooden picks. Place in a baking dish, cover, and bake about 15 minutes. Makes 4 servings.

Each serving contains:

Cal.	Cal. from Fat	Protein	Carb.	Total Fiber	Total Fat	Sat. Fat	Chol.	Sodium
185	37	26g	11g	3g	4g	1g	56mg	178mg

Exchanges:

1/2 Bread/Starch, 3 Very Lean Meat/Protein, 1 Vegetable, 1 Fat

Tuna & Pasta

Enjoy this as a main dish for lunch or a light supper.

1/2 cup (115 g) cooked black beans, drained
1 (6-ounce/170-g) can water-packed tuna, drained
2 green onions, chopped
1 small cucumber, thinly sliced
2 tomatoes, chopped
8 green olives, pitted and chopped
4 ounces (114 g) hot cooked mostaccioli pasta
1/3 cup (80 ml) Italian Dressing (page 83)
1 tablespoon chopped fresh parsley

Rinse and drain beans. In a large mixing bowl, combine tuna, beans, green onions, cucumber, tomatoes, and olives. Add hot cooked pasta. Toss all together with Italian Dressing. Serve at once, sprinkled with parsley, or cover and refrigerate 2 hours to chill thoroughly. Makes 4 servings.

Each serving contains:

Cal.	Cal. from Fat	Protein	Carb.	Total Fiber	Total Fat	Sat. Fat	Chol.	Sodium
149	40	14g	17g	3g	5g	0.7g	19mg	490mg

Exchanges:

1 Bread/Starch, 2 Very Lean Meat/Protein, 1 Vegetable, 1 Fat

Meats

Meat is an excellent source of complete protein but, like other foods containing fat, it should be eaten in moderate amounts. For most recipes, a serving is about 3 ounces (85 g). To keep the saturated-fat content low, choose flank or top-round steak when buying beef. I have also included pork in recipes for this chapter. Because of the new methods of feeding, pork is not as fat as it was 20 years ago. Lamb tends to be fattier, so look for lean cuts.

Make it a habit to trim all visible fat from cuts of beef, pork or lamb. For easy slicing, partially freeze meat (boneless poultry, too) before attempting to cut it into thin strips. This is especially helpful when you are preparing stir-fry dishes. You can easily extend ground meat dishes by adding 1/2 cup rice (85 g) or oat bran (40 g) for each pound of meat. If you have leftover steak, slice it thinly and refrigerate. Then create your own chef's salad by combining the chilled meat with vegetables and salad greens.

When you're in the mood for steak, try Marinated Flank Steak, which has a mystery ingredient that enhances the flavor. Beef & Tomato Stir-Fry features a classic blend of Chinese ingredients and the crunch of walnuts. For a Mediterranean twist, you can't beat Lamb Kabobs, which are extra moist, tender and flavorful, thanks to a marinade of seasoned yogurt. When you're entertaining, impress your guests with an easy but elegant entrée of Apricot-Stuffed Pork Tenderloin. And don't wait for St. Patrick's day to try my Corned Beef & Cabbage recipe, which is a variation of one from an Irish friend.

Corned Beef & Cabbage

Whether you serve it hot or chilled, this is an ideal dish for your next party.

3 to 3½ pounds (1.8 kg) brisket of beef
1 (10-ounce/280-g) package frozen boiling onions
3 carrots, sliced
1 medium head green cabbage, cut into wedges

Marinade:
3 garlic cloves
3 tablespoons pickling spice
1 onion, sliced
2 bay leaves
6 cloves
10 whole black peppercorns
1 cup (250 ml) apple juice

Trim all visible fat from beef. Place in a large mixing bowl with marinade. Cover and marinate overnight. Transfer beef and marinade to a large pot, cover with water, and bring to a boil; reduce heat. Cover and simmer until beef is tender, about 3 hours. Remove beef and let stand 15 minutes. Slice and keep warm. Discard bay leaves and whole spices. Add onions, carrots and cabbage to pot. Cover and cook until tender. Serve vegetables with beef. Makes 8 to 10 servings.

Each serving contains:

Cal.	Cal. from Fat	Protein	Carb.	Total Fiber	Total Fat	Sat. Fat	Chol.	Sodium
480	261	40g	14g	3g	29g	11g	129mg	107mg

Exchanges:

5½ Lean Meat/Protein, 2½ Vegetable, 3 Fat

Beef & Tomato Stir-Fry

For best results, partially freeze the steak before slicing it into thin strips

2 teaspoons canola oil
2 garlic cloves
1 tablespoon sliced fresh ginger
1 pound (450 g) lean sirloin steak, thinly sliced
4 green onions, cut into 2-inch (5-cm) pieces
1/2 cup (55 g) sliced water chestnuts
2 tomatoes, cut into 6 wedges
2 tablespoons chopped walnuts
2 teaspoons cornstarch
1 tablespoon reduced-sodium soy sauce
2 tablespoons dry sherry
2 cups cooked white rice (3/4 cup/100 g uncooked)

Heat oil in a wok or large nonstick skillet. Add garlic and ginger and stir-fry until golden; remove and discard. Add steak slices and quickly stir-fry until meat is no longer pink, about 2 minutes. Add green onions, water chestnuts, tomatoes and walnuts. Continue to stir-fry about 1 minute. In a cup, blend cornstarch with soy sauce and sherry; stir to dissolve cornstarch. Pour into wok or skillet, stirring constantly until sauce is slightly thickened and pieces are well coated. Serve over rice. Makes 4 servings.

Each serving contains:

Cal.	Cal. from Fat	Protein	Carb.	Total Fiber	Total Fat	Sat. Fat	Chol.	Sodium
392	99	31g	40g	4g	11g	3g	75mg	237mg

Exchanges:

2 Bread/Starch, 3 Lean Meat/Protein, 2 Vegetable, 1/2 Fat

Chile Beef & Bean Burgers

Chile peppers provide extra flavor, and beans extra fiber.

1/4 cup (55 g) mashed cooked pinto beans
3/4 pound (340 g) extra-lean ground beef
2 green onions, chopped
1/4 cup (55 g) chopped, peeled and roasted green chiles
1 tablespoon low-sodium catsup
1/2 teaspoon chili powder
1 teaspoon dried leaf oregano
4 English muffins or hamburger buns, split
Lettuce

In a medium mixing bowl, combine all ingredients except English muffins and lettuce. Shape into 4 patties. Heat a large nonstick skillet. Place patties in skillet and pan-broil on each side until cooked through. (Patties can also be broiled.) Toast muffins; top with burgers and lettuce. Makes 4 servings.

Each burger contains:

Cal.	Cal. from Fat	Protein	Carb.	Total Fiber	Total Fat	Sat. Fat	Chol.	Sodium
303	80	23g	31g	3g	9g	3g	31mg	432mg

Exchanges:

2 Bread/Starch, 2½ Lean Meat/Protein, 1/2 Fat

Hamburgers Supreme

The secret to keeping these hamburgers juicy is putting the condiments inside *the hamburger.*

2 green onions, chopped
1 teaspoon Dijon-style mustard
1 tablespoon sweet pickle relish
1 tablespoon low-sodium catsup
1/4 teaspoon garlic powder
3/4 pound (340 g) flank steak, ground
1/4 cup (20 g) oat bran
2 hamburger buns
Lettuce
1 tomato, sliced
Black pepper to taste

In a medium mixing bowl, combine green onions, mustard, relish, catsup, garlic powder, beef and oat bran. Thoroughly mix together. Shape into 4 patties. Preheat broiler. Place patties on a broiler pan and broil on each side until cooked through. Lightly toast hamburger buns. Top each bun half with a burger, lettuce leaf and tomato slice. Season to taste with pepper. Makes 4 open-face burgers.

Each burger contains:

Cal.	Cal. from Fat	Protein	Carb.	Total Fiber	Total Fat	Sat. Fat	Chol.	Sodium
289	85	23g	29g	3g	9g	3g	44mg	357mg

Exchanges:

2 Bread/Starch, 2½ Very Lean Meat/Protein, 1½ Fat

Marinated Flank Steak

Challenge your guests to identify the marinade ingredients!

Marinade:
1 teaspoon instant coffee granules
2 tablespoons hot water
1 garlic clove
1/2 teaspoon dry mustard
1/2 teaspoon dried leaf tarragon
1 tablespoon olive oil
2 tablespoons dry vermouth
2 tablespoons lemon juice

1 pound (450 g) flank steak, cut into 4 pieces
1 tablespoon cornstarch

Dissolve coffee granules in hot water. Combine with remaining marinade ingredients. Place steak in a shallow baking dish and pour marinade over it. Cover and refrigerate about 3 hours. Remove steak from marinade and reserve marinade. Spray a large nonstick skillet with vegetable cooking spray. Heat skillet and pan-broil steak until cooked as desired. (Steak can also be broiled.) Dissolve cornstarch in marinade; pour into a small nonstick saucepan and simmer until thickened. Pour over steak. Makes 4 servings.

Each serving contains:

Cal.	Cal. from Fat	Protein	Carb.	Total Fiber	Total Fat	Sat. Fat	Chol.	Sodium
234	110	24g	4g	0g	12g	4g	59mg	74mg

Exchanges:

3 1/2 Very Lean Meat/Protein, 2 1/2 Fat

Sun-Dried Tomato Meat Loaf

Turn an everyday dish into a special treat for dinner. Leftovers make equally special sandwiches.

1½ pounds (675 g) lean ground beef
1/2 onion, chopped
1 celery stalk, chopped
1 egg or equivalent egg substitute
3/4 cup (60 g) quick-cooking rolled oats
2 tablespoons chili sauce
6 dry-pack sun-dried tomatoes, chopped
3 tablespoons chopped fresh parsley
1/4 green bell pepper, chopped
1/4 cup (60 ml) fat-free milk
1 teaspoon garlic powder
1/2 teaspoon black pepper

Preheat oven to 350F (175C). Spray a 9 x 5 inch (23 x 13-cm) loaf pan with vegetable cooking spray. In a bowl, combine all ingredients; do not overmix. Form into a loaf, place in prepared pan, and bake about 1 hour. Pour off excess juices and let stand about 10 minutes before slicing. Makes 8 servings.

Each serving contains:

Cal.	Cal. from Fat	Protein	Carb.	Total Fiber	Total Fat	Sat. Fat	Chol.	Sodium
200	80	20g	9g	2g	9g	3g	58mg	143mg

Exchanges:

1/2 Bread/Starch, 2½ Lean Meat/Protein, 1/2 Vegetable, 1½ Fat

Beef Pot Roast

Don't try to hurry this dish; slow cooking assures a tender result.

3/4 pound (340 g) boneless chuck or rump roast
1 onion, chopped
2 garlic cloves, minced
1 teaspoon dried leaf sage
2 cups (500 ml) dry red wine
2 carrots, sliced
2 celery stalks, sliced
2 tomatoes, peeled and chopped
2 tablespoons chopped fresh parsley

Spray a Dutch oven or heavy pot with olive oil cooking spray. Heat Dutch oven and brown meat on all sides. Add onion, garlic, sage and wine. Cover and simmer about 1 1/2 hours, turning meat 2 times during cooking and adding water if needed. Add carrots, celery, tomatoes and parsley; cook 30 minutes longer or until vegetables are tender. Makes 6 to 8 servings.

Each serving contains:

Cal.	Cal. from Fat	Protein	Carb.	Total Fiber	Total Fat	Sat. Fat	Chol.	Sodium
216	86	12g	8g	2g	10g	4g	39mg	53mg

Exchanges:

1 1/2 Lean Meat/Protein, 1 1/2 Vegetable, 1 1/2 Fat

Lamb Stew

White wine helps to tenderize the meat while also adding subtle flavor.

3 tablespoons all-purpose flour
2 teaspoons sweet paprika
1/2 teaspoon black pepper
1 pound (450 g) boneless lamb, cut into 1-inch (2.5 cm) cubes
1 tablespoon olive oil
1 garlic clove, minced
1½ cups (185 g) frozen whole onions
2 celery stalks, sliced
2 carrots, sliced
3 all-purpose potatoes, peeled and cubed
2 tomatoes, peeled, seeded and chopped
2 cups (500 ml) water
1/2 cup (120 ml) dry white wine or vermouth
1 cup (115 g) fresh or frozen peas
1/3 cup (85 g) plain nonfat yogurt

In a bowl, stir together 2 tablespoons flour, paprika and pepper. Dredge meat in flour mixture, coating all pieces. Heat oil in a nonstick Dutch oven or large heavy pot. Brown meat on all sides. Add garlic, onions, celery, carrots, potatoes, tomatoes, water and wine. Bring to a boil, cover, reduce heat, and simmer about 45 minutes. Add peas and cook another 5 minutes. Remove meat and vegetables to a serving bowl; cover. Stir remaining 1 tablespoon flour into yogurt to make a paste. Stir paste into remaining stew liquid to make a gravy, adding more water if necessary. Pour over meat and vegetables. Serve at once. Makes 6 servings.

Each serving contains:

Cal.	Cal. from Fat	Protein	Carb.	Total Fiber	Total Fat	Sat. Fat	Chol.	Sodium
378	154	23g	30g	4g	17g	6g	72mg	86mg

Exchanges:

1½ Bread/Starch, 2½ Lean Meat/Protein, 1½ Vegetable, 2 Fat

Lamb Kabobs

For a more intense flavor, refrigerate lamb in marinade for 2 days before cooking.

1/2 cup (115 g) plain nonfat yogurt
1/8 teaspoon ground cinnamon
1/8 teaspoon ground cloves
2 teaspoons chopped fresh parsley
1 tablespoon lemon juice
1/2 teaspoon dried onion flakes
1/2 teaspoon fines herbes
1 1/2 pounds (675 g) boneless leg of lamb, trimmed and
    cut into 1-inch (2.5-cm) cubes
18 cherry tomatoes
2 green bell peppers, cut into cubes
1 onion, cut into 16 pieces

In a large mixing bowl, combine yogurt, cinnamon, cloves, parsley, lemon juice, onion flakes and fines herbes. Add lamb and stir to coat all pieces. Cover and refrigerate 4 hours or overnight. Preheat broiler. Thread lamb cubes, cherry tomatoes, bell peppers and onion onto skewers. Broil, turning several times, until meat is cooked as desired. Makes 6 servings.

Each serving contains:

Cal.	Cal. from Fat	Protein	Carb.	Total Fiber	Total Fat	Sat. Fat	Chol.	Sodium
189	59	25g	7g	1g	7g	2g	73mg	73mg

Exchanges:

3 1/2 Very Lean Meat/Protein, 1 Vegetable, 1 1/2 Fat

Pork Chops with Apples

When pan-broiling, be careful not to overcook the meat, or it will be tough.

4 loin pork chops, about 1⁄ pounds (565 g) total
2 apples, peeled, cored and sliced
1/2 onion, sliced
1/2 teaspoon ground cinnamon
2/3 cup (160 ml) apple juice

In a large nonstick skillet, brown chops quickly on both sides. Add remaining ingredients. Cover, reduce heat, and simmer until apples and onions are tender. Serve chops topped with apples and onions. Makes 4 servings.

Each serving contains:

Cal.	Cal. from Fat	Protein	Carb.	Total Fiber	Total Fat	Sat. Fat	Chol.	Sodium
189	46	18g	17g	3g	5g	2g	52mg	40mg

Exchanges:

2fi Very Lean Meat/Protein, 1 Fruit, 1 Fat

Apricot-Stuffed Pork Tenderloin

Ideal for that special Sunday dinner, served with steamed broccoli and Red Cabbage Slaw, page 64.

1 teaspoon grated orange zest
1 teaspoon dry mustard
1/2 teaspoon dried leaf thyme
1/2 teaspoon paprika
1/2 teaspoon garlic powder
1 pound (450 g) trimmed boneless pork tenderloin
8 to 10 dried apricots
2 tablespoons low-sugar orange marmalade

Preheat oven to 350F (175C). In a cup, stir together orange zest, mustard, thyme, paprika and garlic powder. Cut tenderloin horizontally almost in half, leaving one long side connected. Open tenderloin and lay flat; sprinkle with three-quarters of zest mixture. Place apricots in a row down center of one half of tenderloin. Lift other half over apricots and secure by tying with string at 2-inch (5-cm) intervals, making a firm roll. Place on a baking rack; sprinkle remaining zest mixture on top, patting it in. Roast about 40 minutes. Spread marmalade over top; continue roasting 15 to 20 minutes. Remove from oven, cover with foil, and let rest for 10 minutes before slicing. Makes 4 servings.

Each serving contains:

Cal.	Cal. from Fat	Protein	Carb.	Total Fiber	Total Fat	Sat. Fat	Chol.	Sodium
218	72	25g	11g	1g	8g	3g	68mg	47mg

Exchanges:

3½ Very Lean Meat/Protein, 1 Fruit, 1½ Fat

Pork & Broccoli Stir-Fry

No need to go out for Chinese food. You can prepare this colorful dish at home easily.

Marinade:
1 tablespoon reduced-sodium soy sauce

1 teaspoon sugar

1 teaspoon cornstarch

1 teaspoon grated fresh ginger

1 pound (450 g) pork tenderloin, sliced into thin strips

1 pound (450 g) broccoli crowns

2 tablespoons vegetable oil

1 garlic clove

2 green onions, cut into 2-inch (5-cm) lengths

1/4 cup (60 ml) water

2 1/2 cups cooked white rice (125 g uncooked)

In a bowl, combine marinade ingredients. Add pork and mix well, set aside for 15 minutes. Break or cut flowerets off broccoli and slice stems; set aside. Heat oil in a wok or large skillet; add garlic and pork. Stir-fry about 3 minutes; remove meat. Add broccoli, green onions and water to wok; cook about 3 minutes. Return pork to wok, cover, and cook until water evaporates. Broccoli will be tender-crisp. Serve at once over rice. Makes 6 servings.

Each serving contains:

Cal.	Cal. from Fat	Protein	Carb.	Total Fiber	Total Fat	Sat. Fat	Chol.	Sodium
272	68	20g	31g	3g	8g	2g	49mg	160mg

Exchanges:

1 1/2 Bread/Starch, 2 1/2 Very Lean Meat/Protein, 1 Vegetable, 1 1/2 Fat

Poultry

Several recipes in this chapter combine chicken with fruit or fruit juice. If this is a new concept to you, try Chicken with Peaches and enjoy the refreshing flavor combination. In fact, a variety of tempting flavorings in these recipes, such as Chinese five-spice in Mandarin Chicken, give poultry sensational taste while keeping down fat. Remember that removing the skin removes much of poultry's fat.

When shopping for poultry, compare the per-pound pricing. Poultry skin and bones account for 60 to 70% of the total weight. Sometimes boned, skinned chicken may seem higher priced but actually costs less for the edible portion and will save you a lot of work.

Be guided in your purchase of poultry by the type of cooking you do. If you like to make soups and salads, the whole chicken may be your choice. Bone out the breasts and refrigerate or freeze for later use in recipes. Cook the remaining chicken to make stock for soup and the meat for salads or sandwiches.

Always remove the skin and any visible fat from poultry. If you are concerned that skinned, boned poultry will be too dry, be careful not to overcook it. I think that marinating helps to keep poultry moist, as well as tenderizing it. Marinades can be as simple as bottled Italian dressing, barbecue sauce or yogurt. Braising chicken is an easy, fast cooking method that also helps to seal in moisture.

Because ovens differ so much, when baking poultry, check for doneness about 10 minutes before the time suggested in a recipe. Boneless, skinless pieces can overcook very easily. When cooking Grilled Chile Chicken, turn pieces often to assure even cooking.

Personalize the recipes here as you choose by using different vegetables, fruits, or seasonings. And remember that you can easily substitute chicken and turkey for other meats in many recipes.

Grilled Chile Chicken

Perk up the flavor of chicken with a true taste of the Southwest.

2 tablespoons lemon juice
1/2 teaspoon dried leaf oregano
1/4 teaspoon paprika
1 pound (450 g) skinned and boned chicken breasts
2 teaspoons canola oil
1/4 cup (30 g) chopped onion
1 garlic clove, chopped
1 roasted green chile, peeled and chopped
1 tomato, chopped
3 ounces (85 g) part-skim mozzarella cheese, thinly sliced
1 tablespoon chopped fresh cilantro

Mix lemon juice, oregano and paprika. Pour over chicken, turning pieces to coat; refrigerate 1 hour or more. Preheat broiler. Heat oil in a small nonstick skillet. Add onion and garlic; sauté until softened, not browned. Add chiles and tomatoes, and cook 3 to 4 minutes; cover and set aside. Broil chicken pieces on both sides until done. Remove broiler pan, lay cheese slices on top of chicken, and spoon chile mixture over all. Return to broiler until cheese melts. Sprinkle with cilantro and serve at once. Makes 4 servings.

Each serving contains:

Cal.	Cal. from Fat	Protein	Carb.	Total Fiber	Total Fat	Sat. Fat	Chol.	Sodium
206	89	24g	4g	1g	10g	2g	73mg	83mg

Exchanges:

3½ Very Lean Meat/Protein, 1 Vegetable, 2 Fat

Chicken Cilantro

Spicy Green Beans, page 114, is a good accompaniment.

1 pound (450 g) skinned and boned chicken pieces
1/2 teaspoon paprika
2 teaspoons olive oil
1/2 cup (120 ml) orange juice
1 tomato, chopped
2 green onions, chopped
4 tablespoons chopped fresh cilantro or parsley

Sprinkle chicken pieces with paprika, patting it in. Heat oil in a medium nonstick skillet and brown chicken. Add remaining ingredients. Cover, reduce heat, and cook about 15 minutes, turning chicken at least twice. Makes 4 servings.

Each serving contains:

Cal.	Cal. from Fat	Protein	Carb.	Total Fiber	Total Fat	Sat. Fat	Chol.	Sodium
197	766	24g	6g	1g	8g	2g	72mg	74mg

Exchanges:

3½ Very Lean Meat/Protein, 1/2 Fruit, 1½ Fat

Chicken Italiano

Choose your favorite pasta for this extra-easy dish.

3/4 pound (340 g) skinned and boned chicken pieces
2 green onions, chopped
1/2 cup (120 ml) low-sodium tomato sauce
2 tablespoons chopped sun-dried tomatoes
1/4 cup (60 ml) red wine
2 tablespoons chopped fresh parsley
8 ounces (230 g) macaroni, cooked

Spray a medium nonstick skillet with olive oil cooking spray. Heat skillet and brown chicken. Move pieces aside and stir-fry green onions about 1 minute. Remove skillet from heat and stir in remaining ingredients except pasta. Cover and simmer until chicken is done, about 15 minutes. Serve over cooked pasta. Makes 4 servings.

Each serving contains:

Cal.	Cal. from Fat	Protein	Carb.	Total Fiber	Total Fat	Sat. Fat	Chol.	Sodium
223	45	21g	20g	1g	5g	1g	54mg	95mg

Exchanges:

1 Bread/Starch, 2 1/2 Very Lean Meat/Protein, 1 Vegetable, 1 Fat

Mandarin Chicken

Five-spice powder is a blend of star anise, cinnamon, cloves, fennel (sweet anise) and Szechuan peppercorns.

2 teaspoons canola oil
3/4 pound (340 g) skinned and boned chicken pieces
1 tablespoon reduced-sodium soy sauce
1/2 teaspoon Chinese five-spice powder
2/3 cup (160 ml) fat-free chicken broth or rice wine

Heat oil in a medium nonstick skillet. Add chicken and sauté until browned. Remove skillet from heat. Add soy sauce and sprinkle with five-spice powder. Add broth or rice wine. Cook 5 to 7 minutes, covered. Turn chicken, cover and cook 8 to 10 minutes longer. Makes 4 servings.

Variation

Substitute 1 tablespoon Worcestershire sauce for soy sauce and apple juice for broth. Add 1 apple, peeled, cored and cut into 8 wedges.

Each serving contains:

Cal.	Cal. from Fat	Protein	Carb.	Total Fiber	Total Fat	Sat. Fat	Chol.	Sodium
142	63	18g	1g	0g	7g	2g	54mg	220mg

Exchanges:

2½ Very Lean Meat/Protein, 1½ Fat

Chicken with Peaches

Nectarines can be substituted for peaches in this dish, which features an unusual combination of flavors.

1 tablespoon canola oil
1/2 onion, chopped
1 pound (450 g) skinned and boned chicken pieces
1/2 teaspoon garlic powder
1 (6-inch/15-cm) stalk lemongrass
2 cups (500 ml) passion fruit juice
1/4 teaspoon chili powder
1 tablespoon cornstarch
2 large peaches, peeled, pitted and sliced
4 teaspoons chopped fresh cilantro or parsley, for garnish

Heat oil in a medium nonstick skillet. Add onion and sauté until softened, not browned. Add chicken and lightly brown on all sides. Sprinkle with garlic powder. Crush thick end of lemongrass and add to pan. Pour in 1 cup (250 ml) passion fruit juice and add chili powder. Reduce heat, cover, and cook over medium heat about 15 minutes. Dissolve cornstarch in remaining cup of passion fruit juice. Stir into skillet and cook until slightly thickened. Add peach slices. Cook about 5 minutes. Remove lemongrass. Serve chicken topped with peaches and sauce. Garnish with chopped cilantro. Makes 4 servings.

Each serving contains:

Cal.	Cal. from Fat	Protein	Carb.	Total Fiber	Total Fat	Sat. Fat	Chol.	Sodium
295	86	25g	29g	2g	10g	2g	72mg	80mg

Exchanges:

3 1/2 Very Lean Meat/Protein, 2 Fruit, 2 Fat

Orange Chicken Casserole

Serve with fresh asparagus or green beans.

1 cup (140 g) uncooked long-grain white rice
1/2 cup (120 ml) low-sodium chicken broth
1½ cups (375 ml) orange juice
2 tablespoons dried currants
2 tablespoons chopped pistachios
3/4 pound (340 g) skinned and boned chicken breasts
1/2 cup (115 g) plain nonfat yogurt
1/2 teaspoon dried leaf tarragon
Paprika
1 (11-ounce/310-g) can Mandarin oranges, drained

Preheat oven to 350F (175C). Spread rice evenly over bottom of a 2-quart (2-liter) baking dish. Combine chicken broth, orange juice, currants and pistachios in a small mixing bowl. Pour over rice. Place chicken breasts on top. Brush chicken with yogurt. Sprinkle with tarragon and paprika. Cover and bake about 30 minutes; uncover, add Mandarin oranges, and continue baking about 15 minutes or until chicken is done. Makes 4 servings.

Each serving contains:

Cal.	Cal. from Fat	Protein	Carb.	Total Fiber	Total Fat	Sat. Fat	Chol.	Sodium
379	34	27g	59g	2g	4g	1g	51mg	107mg

Exchanges:

2 Bread/Starch, 3 Very Lean Meat/Protein, 1½ Fruit, 1 Fat

Baked Rosemary Chicken

Serve hot for an evening meal, or chill and take along for a superb picnic.

2 pounds (900 g) chicken pieces, skinned
1/2 cup (7 g) crushed shredded wheat cereal
1 teaspoon crushed dried leaf rosemary
1½ teaspoons paprika
1 tablespoon grated orange zest
1 teaspoon dried leaf oregano
3/4 cup (180 ml) evaporated skimmed milk

Preheat oven to 375F (190C). Spray a baking sheet with vegetable cooking spray. Remove all visible fat from chicken. Combine cereal, rosemary, paprika, orange zest and oregano in a pie plate or small paper bag. Pour evaporated milk into another pie plate. Dip each chicken piece into milk and then into cereal mixture. Place coated pieces on prepared baking sheet. Bake 30 to 40 minutes. Makes 6 servings.

Each serving contains:

Cal.	Cal. from Fat	Protein	Carb.	Total Fiber	Total Fat	Sat. Fat	Chol.	Sodium
246	74	34g	7g	1g	8g	2g	97mg	130mg

Exchanges:

4½ Very Lean Meat/Protein, 1/2 Skim Milk, 1½ Fat

Chicken in Salsa Verde

Fresh tomatillos resemble green tomatoes but have a papery husk. If you can't find fresh tomatillos, the canned variety is a fine substitute.

2 teaspoons canola oil
1 pound (450 g) skinned and boned chicken pieces
1/2 onion, chopped
1 garlic clove, minced
1 pound (450 g) fresh or 1 (12-ounce/340-g) can tomatillos, drained
3 whole roasted green chilies, peeled and chopped
1/2 cup (120 ml) apple juice
1 tablespoon chopped fresh cilantro

Spray a large nonstick skillet with vegetable cooking spray. Heat oil and sauté chicken on all sides until lightly browned. Add onion and garlic, stirring until limp. Add remaining ingredients. Reduce heat, cover, and simmer about 20 minutes. Makes 4 servings.

Each serving contains:

Cal.	Cal. from Fat	Protein	Carb.	Total Fiber	Total Fat	Sat. Fat	Chol.	Sodium
243	85	25g	15g	3g	9g	2g	72mg	75mg

Exchanges:

3 1/2 Very Lean Meat/Protein, 3 Vegetable, 2 Fat

Soft Chicken Tacos

No frying needed. For authentic south-of-the-border tacos, just heat and fill soft corn tortillas.

2 teaspoons canola oil
1/4 onion, chopped
1 cup (170 g) chopped cooked chicken
8 corn tortillas
1 cup (230 g) Tomato Salsa (page 91)
1/2 cup (55 g) shredded low-fat Monterey Jack cheese
1 cup (70 g) shredded lettuce
12 radishes, sliced

In a 2-quart (2-liter) nonstick saucepan, heat oil and sauté onion until softened, not browned. Add chicken, cover, and heat through. Warm tortillas in oven or microwave oven. Spoon chicken mixture on each tortilla and top with salsa, cheese, lettuce and radishes. Fold in half and serve. Makes 8 tacos.

Each taco contains:

Cal.	Cal. from Fat	Protein	Carb.	Total Fiber	Total Fat	Sat. Fat	Chol.	Sodium
134	40	9g	15g	2g	4g	1g	21mg	255mg

Exchanges:

1 Bread/Starch, 1 Very Lean Meat/Protein, 1/2 Vegetable, 1 Fat

Turkey Chili

Avid chili fans may want to increase the amount of chili powder.

1 tablespoon canola oil
1 pound (450 g) ground turkey
1 onion, chopped
1 garlic clove, crushed
3 large tomatoes, peeled and chopped
1 (8-ounce/230-g) can low-sodium tomato sauce
1 tablespoon chili powder
1 tablespoon chopped fresh oregano or
   1 teaspoon dried leaf oregano
1 tablespoons chopped fresh cilantro
1/2 teaspoon ground cumin
1 (14 1/2-ounce/415-g) can pinto or kidney beans, drained
1/4 cup (55 g) plain nonfat yogurt
2 tablespoons chopped fresh cilantro, for garnish

Heat oil in a 5 1/2-quart (5.5-liter) nonstick saucepan. Add turkey and stir until crumbled and browned. Add onion, garlic, tomatoes, tomato sauce, chili powder, oregano, cilantro and cumin. Cover and cook over low heat for 1 hour. Add drained pinto or kidney beans. Cover and heat through. Spoon into individual bowls. Top each serving with yogurt and additional cilantro. Makes 6 servings.

Each serving contains:

Cal.	Cal. from Fat	Protein	Carb.	Total Fiber	Total Fat	Sat. Fat	Chol.	Sodium
274	93	22g	25g	9g	10g	2g	55mg	89mg

Exchanges:

1 Bread/Starch, 2 1/2 Very Lean Meat/Protein, 1 1/2 Vegetable, 1 Fat

Chicken-Chile Sandwich

For a quick, tasty lunch, serve with colorful Three Bell-Pepper Salad,
page 76.

2 slices sourdough bread
2 teaspoons Dijon-style mustard
1 tablespoon Green Chile Mayonnaise (page 86)
2 lettuce leaves
3 ounces (85 g) sliced cooked chicken
1 tomato, sliced
2 roasted green chiles, peeled and seeded
1/2 avocado, peeled and thinly sliced

Lightly toast bread. Spread each slice of toasted bread with
mustard and with Green Chile Mayonnaise. Top with lettuce,
sliced chicken, tomato, a green chile and avocado. Makes
2 servings.

Each sandwich contains:

Cal.	Cal. from Fat	Protein	Carb.	Total Fiber	Total Fat	Sat. Fat	Chol.	Sodium
268	111	17g	24g	5g	12g	2g	38mg	329mg

Exchanges:

1 Bread/Starch, 1½ Very Lean Meat/Protein, 2 Vegetable, 2 Fat

Deviled Turkey Pita Pockets

This filling can serve as a salad as well as a sandwich.

1 cup (170 g) chopped cooked turkey
1/4 cup (30 g) chopped celery
1 green onion, chopped
2 tablespoons chopped sweet pickle
1 tablespoon chopped pimiento
1/2 teaspoon prepared horseradish
1/2 teaspoon Dijon-style mustard
2 tablespoons plain nonfat yogurt
4 whole wheat pita bread pockets
12 cherry tomatoes, halved
1 cucumber, sliced
4 lettuce leaves, shredded

In a small mixing bowl, combine turkey, celery, green onion, pickle, pimiento, horseradish, mustard and yogurt. Cut pitas in half, open pocket, and fill with turkey mixture, cherry tomatoes, cucumber and lettuce. Makes 4 servings.

Each sandwich contains:

Cal.	Cal. from Fat	Protein	Carb.	Total Fiber	Total Fat	Sat. Fat	Chol.	Sodium
270	35	18g	44g	6g	4g	1g	27mg	490mg

Exchanges:

2 1/2 Bread/Starch, 1 1/2 Very Lean Meat/Protein, 1 1/2 Vegetable, 1 Fat

Barbecued Turkey Burgers

For added flavor, brush the burgers with barbecue sauce while broiling.

3/4 pound (340 g) lean ground turkey
1/4 cup (20 g) oat bran or quick-cooking rolled oats
2 tablespoons low-sodium barbecue sauce
1 teaspoon Dijon-style mustard
1 green onion, chopped
4 teaspoons nonfat mayonnaise
4 hamburger buns
4 slices low-fat cheddar cheese
Lettuce

Preheat broiler. In a medium mixing bowl, combine turkey, oat bran or rolled oats, barbecue sauce, mustard and green onion. Shape into 4 burgers. Broil 7 to 10 minutes on each side or until cooked through. Lightly spread mayonnaise on buns. Top with burgers, cheese and lettuce. Makes 4 burgers.

Each burger contains:

Cal.	Cal. from Fat	Protein	Carb.	Total Fiber	Total Fat	Sat. Fat	Chol.	Sodium
342	116	29g	28g	3g	13g	4g	68mg	557mg

Exchanges:

2 Bread/Starch, 3 Lean Meat/Protein, 1 Fat

Desserts

It is possible to look forward to dessert after a lovely meal without feeling guilty. Desserts made with fresh fruits are the stars here because their fresh flavors and bright colors are enticing and most of the recipes are low in fat. Some require a little more preparation time, while picture-pretty Ricotta-Filled Peaches can be prepared in minutes. By combining fruits and berries in Apple-Blackberry Cobbler, the familiar cobbler takes on a new look. Date-Pecan Bread Pudding transforms plain bread into a delicious dessert.

I have not forgotten that chocolate is probably our favorite dessert flavor. By using cocoa powder rather than solid chocolate, which is high in fat, you can still enjoy treats such as Chocolate Mocha Pudding.

My favorite desserts have always been frozen or made with fruit—or both! That craving is satisfied beautifully with Pineapple Sherbet. Most of the time my guests never guess they're eating frozen buttermilk and not ice cream. Try my Watermelon Ice and be prepared to offer seconds.

It is increasingly difficult to buy ripe produce, so plan to purchase fruit while allowing ample time for the fruit to ripen. To speed up the ripening process, place fruit plus one apple in a paper sack. Fold over ends of sack, sealing the contents. The apple naturally produces a gas that hastens ripening of the other fruit.

Chocolate Mocha Pudding

This pudding is so rich and creamy, you'll never believe it's sin-free.

1/2 cup (120 ml) warm brewed coffee
1/4 cup (57 g) fructose granules
2 tablespoons cornstarch
3 tablespoons unsweetened cocoa powder
1 cup (250 ml) fat-free milk
1 (12-ounce/375-ml) can evaporated skimmed milk
1/2 cup (120 ml) egg substitute
1 teaspoon vanilla extract

In a saucepan, combine coffee, fructose, cornstarch and cocoa powder; stir until well blended. Stirring constantly, slowly pour in fat-free milk, evaporated milk and egg substitute. Continue stirring while cooking over medium heat until bubbling and thickened, about 7 minutes. Remove from heat; stir in vanilla. Pour into serving dishes. Makes 6 servings.

Each serving contains:

Cal.	Cal. from Fat	Protein	Carb.	Total Fiber	Total Fat	Sat. Fat	Chol.	Sodium
131	10	8g	22g	1g	1g	0g	1mg	139mg

Exchanges:

1 Bread/Starch, 1/2 Skim Milk

Baked Lemon Pudding with Raspberries

The perfect dessert for lemon lovers.

1/2 cup (120 ml) egg substitute
1/4 cup (57 g) fructose granules
3/4 cup (180 ml) reduced-fat buttermilk
1 tablespoon cornstarch
1 tablespoon all-purpose flour
2 teaspoons grated lemon zest
3 tablespoons lemon juice
1 cup (145 g) fresh or frozen raspberries
2 tablespoons sugar

Preheat oven to 350F (175C). Butter 6 individual baking dishes or a 9-inch (23-cm) tart pan. In a bowl, combine egg substitute, fructose, buttermilk, cornstarch, flour, lemon zest and lemon juice. Whisk together until thoroughly combined. Pour into prepared baking dishes and place on a baking sheet on middle oven rack. Place a pan of water on lower rack and bake about 25 minutes or until slightly puffed. Cool. In a bowl, combine raspberries and sugar; spoon over cooled puddings. Makes 6 servings.

Each serving contains:

Cal.	Cal. from Fat	Protein	Carb.	Total Fiber	Total Fat	Sat. Fat	Chol.	Sodium
100	10	4g	19g	2g	1g	0g	1mg	70mg

Exchanges:

1 Bread/Starch, 1/2 Very Lean Meat/Protein, 1/2 Fruit

Date-Pecan Bread Pudding

Turn plain leftover bread into a sensational dessert.

2 cups (500 ml) fat-free milk
1 cup (250 ml) egg substitute
2 tablespoons margarine, melted
1/4 cup (55 g) sugar
2 teaspoons orange extract
3 cups (100 g) cubed French bread
1/3 cup (55 g) chopped dates
1/4 cup (30 g) chopped pecans
1 teaspoon ground cinnamon

Preheat oven to 325F (165C). Spray a 6-cup (1.5-liter) baking dish with vegetable cooking spray. In a large bowl, beat together milk, egg substitute, margarine, sugar and orange extract. Add bread cubes, dates and pecans; mix together until all bread cubes are moistened. Pour into prepared baking dish. Sprinkle with cinnamon. Place a large baking pan on lower oven rack. Place baking dish in pan and add 1 inch (2.5 cm) water to larger pan. Bake about 45 minutes. Serve warm or cold. Makes 6 servings.

Each serving contains:

Cal.	Cal. from Fat	Protein	Carb.	Total Fiber	Total Fat	Sat. Fat	Chol.	Sodium
264	86	11g	34g	2g	10g	2g	6mg	311mg

Exchanges:

1 1/2 Bread/Starch, 1 Very Lean Meat/Protein, 1/2 Fruit, 1/2 Skim Milk, 2 Fat

Warm Fruit Compote

An ideal chafing dish or buffet dessert.

1 (16-ounce/450-g) can juice-packed pineapple chunks
1 (16-ounce/450-g) can juice-packed sliced peaches
1 cup (170 g) red seedless grapes
2 tablespoons chopped crystallized ginger
1/4 cup (60 ml) rum
2 tablespoons sliced almonds
6 tablespoons plain nonfat yogurt
Nutmeg

In a chafing dish or saucepan, heat pineapple and peaches with their juice, grapes, ginger and rum until very warm. To serve, spoon fruit and juice into small bowls. Sprinkle with nuts and top with a dollop of yogurt and a dusting of nutmeg. Makes 6 servings.

Each serving contains:

Cal.	Cal. from Fat	Protein	Carb.	Total Fiber	Total Fat	Sat. Fat	Chol.	Sodium
155	15	2g	30g	2g	2g	0g	0mg	19mg

Exchanges:

1/2 Bread/Starch, 1½ Fruit, 1/2 Fat

Ricotta-Stuffed Peaches

Chopped walnuts offer a nice contrast in texture to the cheese filling. This is equally good with plums or nectarines.

1/4 cup (55 g) nonfat ricotta cheese
1/4 cup (55 g) nonfat cream cheese
1 tablespoon orange or lime juice
1 tablespoon grated orange zest
4 fresh peaches, peeled, pitted and halved
4 teaspoons chopped walnuts

In a small bowl, thoroughly combine ricotta cheese, cream cheese, orange juice and orange zest. Place 2 peach halves on each serving plate. Fill each cavity with cheese mixture and sprinkle with chopped walnuts. Makes 4 servings.

Each serving contains:

Cal.	Cal. from Fat	Protein	Carb.	Total Fiber	Total Fat	Sat. Fat	Chol.	Sodium
127	28	5g	22g	4g	3g	1g	6mg	99mg

Exchanges:

1/2 Very Lean Meat/Protein, 1 1/2 Fruit, 1/2 Fat

Apple-Blackberry Cobbler

Today old-fashioned cobblers are enjoying a revival, regularly appearing on restaurant menus.

Topping:
1/2 cup (70 g) all-purpose flour
1/2 cup (40 g) quick-cooking rolled oats
1/4 cup (40 g) brown sugar
4 tablespoons margarine, melted
1/2 teaspoon ground cardamom
1/4 cup (30 g) chopped walnuts

Filling:
1 1/2 pounds (675 g) Granny Smith apples (5 to 6), peeled,
    cored and sliced
1 cup (145 g) fresh or frozen blackberries
2 tablespoons quick-cooking tapioca
1 tablespoon lemon juice
1 teaspoon almond extract

Preheat oven to 425F (220C). Spray an 9-inch (23-cm) square baking dish with vegetable cooking spray. In a medium bowl, combine topping ingredients until mixture is crumbly; set aside. In a large bowl, toss filling ingredients until apples and blackberries are coated. Carefully spoon into prepared baking dish. Sprinkle topping evenly over filling and bake about 25 minutes. Serve warm or cold. Makes 6 servings.

Each serving contains:

Cal.	Cal. from Fat	Protein	Carb.	Total Fiber	Total Fat	Sat. Fat	Chol.	Sodium
285	101	3g	45g	6g	11g	2g	0mg	5mg

Exchanges:

1 1/2 Bread/Starch, 1 1/2 Fruit, 2 Fat

Raspberry-Blueberry Cobbler

A delicious variation is to substitute sliced nectarines or peaches for the raspberries. Mix and match 3 cups of your favorite berries, fresh or frozen.

2 cups (300 g) fresh or frozen raspberries
1 cup (145 g) fresh or frozen blueberries
1/2 cup (100 g) sugar
2 tablespoons quick-cooking tapioca
2 tablespoons orange juice
1/2 cup (40 g) quick-cooking rolled oats
1/2 cup (70 g) all-purpose flour
1 tablespoon sugar
1/4 cup (60 ml) canola oil
1 teaspoon orange extract

Preheat oven to 350F (175C). Spray an 8-inch (20-cm) square baking dish with vegetable cooking spray. If using fresh berries, rinse and thoroughly drain; frozen berries maybe put directly into baking dish. Combine sugar and tapioca and sprinkle over berries. Stir to distribute evenly. Drizzle orange juice over top. In a bowl, combine oats, flour and sugar; stir in oil and orange extract. Sprinkle mixture over berries and bake in preheated oven about 35 minutes or until top is golden brown. Serve warm. Makes 6 servings.

Each serving contains:

Cal.	Cal. from Fat	Protein	Carb.	Total Fiber	Total Fat	Sat. Fat	Chol.	Sodium
266	89	3g	43g	4g	10g	1g	0mg	2mg

Exchanges:

2 Bread/Starch, 1 Fruit, 2 Fat

Broiled Fresh Pineapple Rings

Enjoy this simple dish as dessert or for brunch.

**1 medium fresh pineapple, peeled and sliced into
    8 to 10 rounds
2 tablespoons margarine, melted
1/4 cup (60 ml) rum (optional)
4 tablespoons granulated brown sugar substitute
1/2 teaspoon ground cinnamon
1/4 teaspoon ground nutmeg**

Preheat broiler or grill. Place pineapple rounds on a broiler
pan or grill rack. Brush with margarine and rum, if using; top
with brown sugar substitute, cinnamon and nutmeg. Broil
until bubbling and slightly browned. Serve at once. Makes
8 to 10 servings.

Each serving contains:

Cal.	Cal. from Fat	Protein	Carb.	Total Fiber	Total Fat	Sat. Fat	Chol.	Sodium
95	29	0g	17g	1g	3g	1g	0mg	1mg

Exchanges:

1 Fruit, 1/2 Fat

Oranges with Strawberries & Hazelnuts

Simplicity at its best.

3 large navel or blood oranges, peeled and sliced in rounds
3 tablespoons balsamic vinegar
1 cup (145 g) sliced strawberries
2 tablespoons chopped roasted hazelnuts

Fan orange slices on 4 serving plates. Sprinkle with vinegar and top with strawberries and chopped hazelnuts. This may be prepared an hour before serving time. Cover and refrigerate until needed. Makes 4 servings.

Each serving contains:

Cal.	Cal. from Fat	Protein	Carb.	Total Fiber	Total Fat	Sat. Fat	Chol.	Sodium
90	23	2g	17g	4g	3g	0g	0mg	4mg

Exchanges:

1 Fruit, 1/2 Fat

Watermelon Ice

A particularly refreshing way to enjoy this sweet summer fruit.

4 cups (900 g) watermelon cubes (1/4 medium)
1 cup (145 g) strawberries
1 cup (250 ml) orange juice
2 tablespoons sugar

Remove and discard watermelon seeds. In a food processor or blender, puree watermelon cubes in several batches. Slice or purée strawberries. Combine all ingredients and pour into freezer canister. Freeze according to manufacturer's directions. Makes 8 to 10 servings.

Each serving contains:

Cal.	Cal. from Fat	Protein	Carb.	Total Fiber	Total Fat	Sat. Fat	Chol.	Sodium
46	1	1g	13g	1g	0g	0g	0mg	3mg

Exchanges:

1 Fruit

Orange Cake

Perfect for a birthday celebration, this cake has a touch of orange both in the cake and in the frosting.

3/4 cup (150 g) sugar
2/3 cup (140 g) margarine
1/2 cup (120 ml) egg substitute
2½ cups (350 g) cake flour
2 teaspoons baking powder
2/3 cup (160 ml) fat-free milk
1 teaspoon orange extract
2 tablespoons orange juice
1 tablespoon grated orange zest
Cooked Orange Frosting (recipe follows)

Preheat oven to 375F (190C). Line a 13 x 9-inch (33 x 23-cm) baking pan with waxed paper and spray with vegetable cooking spray; set aside. In a mixing bowl, beat sugar and margarine until creamy; beat in egg substitute. In another bowl, combine cake flour and baking powder. In a cup, combine milk, orange extract, orange juice and orange peel. With mixer running, alternately add flour and milk mixtures to margarine mixture. Beat at low speed, scraping sides of bowl as necessary. Pour batter into prepared pan; bake about 25 minutes. Cool for 5 minutes. If desired, remove cake from pan and cover with frosting, or frost cake in pan when completely cooled. Makes 12 servings.

Cooked Orange Frosting

5 tablespoons all-purpose flour
1 cup (250 ml) fat-free milk
2/3 cup (140 g) sugar
1/2 cup (115 g) margarine
1½ teaspoons orange extract
1 tablespoon grated orange zest

In a saucepan, blend flour and milk. Stirring constantly, cook over medium heat until mixture thickens, about 3 minutes. Set aside and cool. In a small mixer bowl, beat together sugar and margarine; add orange extract and orange zest. Beat in milk mixture until thoroughly combined and smooth. For best results, refrigerate about 1 hour before spreading on cake. Makes frosting for 1 (13 x 9-inch) or 2 (8-inch) layers.

Each serving of cake contains:

Cal.	Cal. from Fat	Protein	Carb.	Total Fiber	Total Fat	Sat. Fat	Chol.	Sodium
257	96	4g	36g	1g	11g	2g	0mg	65mg

Exchanges:

2 Bread/Starch, 2 Fat

Each serving of frosting contains:

Cal.	Cal. from Fat	Protein	Carb.	Total Fiber	Total Fat	Sat. Fat	Chol.	Sodium
131	69	1g	15g	0g	8g	1g	0mg	99mg

Exchanges:

1 Bread/Starch, 1½ Fat

Pineapple Sherbet

Buttermilk and pineapple make a tangy, pleasing combination in this tropical treat.

2 cups (500 ml) reduced-fat buttermilk
1 (8-ounce/230-g) can juice-packed pineapple chunks
2 teaspoons rum flavoring
1/4 cup (55 g) sugar

Combine all ingredients, including pineapple juice, in a food processor or blender; process until well blended. Pour into freezer canister. Freeze according to manufacturer's directions. Makes 8 to 10 servings.

Each serving contains:

Cal.	Cal. from Fat	Protein	Carb.	Total Fiber	Total Fat	Sat. Fat	Chol.	Sodium
64	6	2g	12g	0g	1g	0g	4mg	65mg

Exchanges:

1/2 Bread/Starch, 1/2 Skim Milk

Crêpes with Cottage-Cheese Filling

These delicate dessert pancakes can be made ahead, covered, and refrigerated until needed.

Crêpe Batter:
1 egg
2 egg whites
1½ cups (375 ml) fat-free milk
1 cup (200 g) all-purpose flour
1 teaspoon vanilla extract
1 teaspoon vegetable oil
2 teaspoons sugar

Cottage-Cheese Filling:
2 cups (450 g) nonfat cottage cheese
1/4 cup (55 g) fat-free sour cream
1 tablespoon sugar
1 teaspoon vanilla extract
1 tablespoon grated lemon zest
2 cups (300 g) sliced fresh strawberries

Crêpes: In a blender, food processor, or bowl, process batter ingredients until well blended. Lightly spray a crêpe pan or small skillet with vegetable cooking spray. Pour about 2 tablespoons batter in pan; immediately tilt pan to swirl batter to cover pan bottom. Cook until surface looks dry and edges are lacy and brown. Turn crêpe over and cook briefly; flip onto a warm plate. Makes 12 crêpes.

Cottage-Cheese Filling: In a small bowl, combine all filling ingredients except strawberries. To fill crêpes, place a heaping tablespoon of filling in center of crêpe, spoon a few strawberries on top; roll one edge over filling, making a cylinder. Top with additional strawberries. Makes filling for 12 crêpes.

Each 2-crêpe serving contains:

Cal.	Cal. from Fat	Protein	Carb.	Total Fiber	Total Fat	Sat. Fat	Chol.	Sodium
109	10	8g	16g	1g	1g	0g	20mg	202mg

Exchanges:

1 Bread/Starch, 1 Very Lean Meat/Protein

Snacks

Snacking is encouraged for the person with borderline diabetes to help maintain an even blood-sugar level. When possible, try to combine a protein and a carbohydrate in your snack; for instance, a pear and a few peanuts; an apple and a thin slice of cheese; air-popped corn with a sprinkle of grated Parmesan cheese.

For midmorning or after-school snacking, whip up a batch of Three-Fruit Bon Bons or Chocolate Peanut Butter Cookies. They're satisfying—eat them without guilt! Trail Mix is a welcome snack at any time of day. It's ideal to keep handy in a little plastic bag. For something more substantial, an open-face sandwich with cream cheese fills the need. Be prepared by keeping a supply of plain bagels, English muffins, puffed rice and corn cakes, and, of course, peanut butter on hand.

Everyone seems to like Cereal Party Mix, which is crunchy and satisfying. The recipe makes about 8 cups and keeps well. Store in a container with a tight-fitting lid or in sealed plastic bags. If you crave a snack while watching a movie, feast on your own Caramel Popcorn. If you prefer a drink, try one of the yogurt smoothies found in the breakfast chapter.

Trail Mix

A snack to take with you; especially good in the car.

1 cup (7 g) air-popped corn
1/4 cup (30 g) dry-roasted peanuts
1/2 cup (75 g) chopped dried apples
1/4 cup (30 g) chopped dates
1/4 cup (30 g) chopped walnuts
1/4 cup (30 g) sunflower seeds

Mix all ingredients together and store in a covered container or a sealed plastic bag. Makes about 7 (1/2-cup) servings.

Each serving contains:

Cal.	Cal. from Fat	Protein	Carb.	Total Fiber	Total Fat	Sat. Fat	Chol.	Sodium
121	67	4g	12g	2g	7g	1g	0mg	6mg

Exchanges:

1/2 Bread/Starch, 1/2 Lean Meat/Protein, 1/2 Fruit, 1 Fat

Cereal Party Mix

A slightly different–and more healthful–version of an all-time favorite.

> **3 tablespoons margarine**
> **1½ teaspoons garlic powder**
> **1/2 teaspoon chili powder**
> **1/4 teaspoon onion powder**
> **1 tablespoon Worcestershire sauce**
> **1 cup (50 g) Wheat Chex**
> **2 cups (60 g) Corn Chex**
> **2 cups (60 g) Crispix**
> **1 cup (30 g) Cheerios**
> **1 cup (60 g) pretzel sticks**
> **1 cup (7 g) air-popped corn**
> **1/2 cup (60 g) mixed dry-roasted nuts**

Heat oven to 250F (120C). Melt margarine in a large baking pan. Stir in garlic powder, chili powder, onion powder and Worcestershire sauce. Add remaining ingredients, and toss to coat all evenly. Bake about 20 minutes, stirring occasionally. Cool and store in a sealed container. Makes about 16 (1/2-cup) servings.

Each serving contains:

Cal.	Cal. from Fat	Protein	Carb.	Total Fiber	Total Fat	Sat. Fat	Chol.	Sodium
118	44	2g	17g	1g	5g	1g	0mg	232mg

Exchanges:

1 Bread/Starch, 1 Fat

Caramel Popcorn

Don't wait for a movie to enjoy this popcorn.

10 cups (70 g) air-popped corn
2 tablespoons honey
3 tablespoons granulated sugar
3 tablespoons brown sugar
1 tablespoon water
2 teaspoons margarine
1 teaspoon vanilla extract

Preheat oven to 300F (150C). Line a baking sheet with foil. Spread popped corn on baking sheet and place in oven while making syrup. In a saucepan, combine remaining ingredients and cook about 5 minutes. Remove popped corn and pour syrup over; mix quickly to coat evenly. Spread out on baking sheet and return to oven. Bake about 15 minutes. Stir and bake another 10 minutes. Break into pieces and store in a covered container. Makes 10 (1-cup) servings.

Each serving contains:

Cal.	Cal. from Fat	Protein	Carb.	Total Fiber	Total Fat	Sat. Fat	Chol.	Sodium
81	10	1g	18g	1g	1g	0g	0mg	2mg

Exchanges:

1 Bread/Starch

Herb-Cheese Popcorn

Here is a savory popcorn for those who don't care for a sweet coating.

10 cups (70 g) air-popped corn
1/2 teaspoon garlic powder
1 teaspoon Italian seasoning
1/2 teaspoon chili powder
2 tablespoons margarine, melted
3 tablespoons grated Parmesan cheese

Place popped corn in a large bowl. Sprinkle with remaining ingredients and toss to coat. Makes 10 (1-cup) servings.

Each serving contains:

Cal.	Cal. from Fat	Protein	Carb.	Total Fiber	Total Fat	Sat. Fat	Chol.	Sodium
60	29	2g	6g	1g	3g	1g	1mg	3mg

Exchanges:

1/2 Bread/Starch, 1/2 Fat

Chocolate Peanut Butter Cookies

Children will have fun making these no-bake cookies.

1 cup (100 g) graham cracker crumbs (12 cookies)
1 tablespoon margarine, melted
1/3 cup (85 g) peanut butter
2 tablespoons chocolate syrup
1 teaspoon orange extract
1 tablespoon fat-free milk
2 tablespoons unsweetened cocoa powder

In a bowl, thoroughly combine all ingredients except cocoa powder. Put cocoa powder in a small deep bowl. Form graham cracker mixture into 1-inch (2.5-cm) balls and roll each ball in cocoa powder. Place on a plate and chill. Makes 18 cookies.

Each cookie contains:

Cal.	Cal. from Fat	Protein	Carb.	Total Fiber	Total Fat	Sat. Fat	Chol.	Sodium
69	34	2g	8g	1g	4g	1g	0mg	65mg

Exchanges:

1/2 Bread/Starch, 1/2 Fat

Three-Fruit Bonbons

If you don't have a food processor, finely chop the fruits and nuts by hand.

1 tablespoon peanut butter
1 tablespoon apple juice
1 tablespoon honey
1/3 cup (55 g) raisins
1/3 cup (55 g) dates
1/3 cup (55 g) prunes
1/3 cup (45 g) walnuts
1 tablespoon sunflower seeds
2 tablespoons powdered sugar

In a bowl, combine peanut butter, apple juice and honey. Combine raisins, dates, prunes, walnuts and sunflower seeds in a food processor and process briefly to chop mixture. Combine the two mixtures in a bowl by hand or in a food processor. Shape into 1-inch (2.5-cm) balls. Place powdered sugar in a small deep bowl; roll balls in sugar to coat. Place on a plate. Makes 12 cookies.

Each cookie contains:

Cal.	Cal. from Fat	Protein	Carb.	Total Fiber	Total Fat	Sat. Fat	Chol.	Sodium
60	25	1g	9g	1g	3g	0g	0mg	9mg

Exchanges:

1/2 Fruit, 1/2 Fat

Broiled Banana Muffin

Satisfyingly sweet and easy to make, this muffin supplies a quick pick-me-up in the afternoon.

2 English muffins, sliced in half
4 teaspoons nonfat cream cheese
1/4 teaspoon ground cinnamon
1 banana, thinly sliced
2 teaspoons honey

Preheat broiler. Toast muffins and remove from broiler. Spread each muffin with a thin layer of cream cheese and sprinkle with cinnamon. Arrange banana slices on top and drizzle with honey. Return to broiler until lightly browned. Makes 4 servings.

Each muffin half contains:

Cal.	Cal. from Fat	Protein	Carb.	Total Fiber	Total Fat	Sat. Fat	Chol.	Sodium
110	7	3g	23g	2g	1g	0g	0mg	159mg

Exchanges:

1 Bread/Starch, 1/2 Fruit

Cheese & Turkey Snack

This open-face snack won't spoil your appetite.

8 teaspoons nonfat cream cheese
8 sesame-seed water crackers
1 tomato, sliced
8 (1-ounce/30-g) slices cooked turkey
1/2 teaspoon dried leaf oregano

Spread cream cheese thinly on each cracker. Top with a tomato slice and a turkey slice. Sprinkle with oregano. Makes 4 servings.

Each serving contains:

Cal.	Cal. from Fat	Protein	Carb.	Total Fiber	Total Fat	Sat. Fat	Chol.	Sodium
135	52	15g	6g	1g	6g	1g	38mg	140mg

Exchanges:

1/2 Bread/Starch, 2 Very Lean Meat/Protein, 1 Fat

Stuffed Celery Sticks

*Make these in the morning and refrigerate in plastic storage bags
until snack time.*

> **1 (3-ounce/85-g) package nonfat cream cheese**
> **1 tablespoon chopped walnuts**
> **2 tablespoons drained crushed pineapple**
> **8 (4-inch/10-cm) celery sticks**

In a small bowl, blend together cream cheese, walnuts and
pineapple. Spread on celery sticks. Refrigerate until needed.
Makes 4 servings.

Each serving contains:

Cal.	Cal. from Fat	Protein	Carb.	Total Fiber	Total Fat	Sat. Fat	Chol.	Sodium
42	13	4g	4g	1g	1g	0g	2mg	151mg

Exchanges:

1/2 Very Lean Meat/Protein, 1 Vegetable

Tuna Dip

Serve with crisp crackers and fresh vegetable sticks.

1 (7-ounce/200-g) can water-packed tuna, drained
2 tablespoons nonfat mayonnaise
1/4 teaspoon dry mustard
1/4 cup (55 g) low-fat cottage cheese
1 green onion, chopped
2 tablespoons chopped celery
1 tablespoon lemon juice
1/2 teaspoon curry powder

In a small bowl, mix all ingredients together. Use as a dip or sandwich filling. Makes about 1½ cups.

Each 2-tablespoon serving contains:

Cal.	Cal. from Fat	Protein	Carb.	Total Fiber	Total Fat	Sat. Fat	Chol.	Sodium
14	2	2g	0g	0g	0g	0g	4mg	41mg

Exchanges:

Free

Stuffed Eggs

A tasty and satisfying after-school snack.

6 eggs
3 tablespoons nonfat mayonnaise
1/2 teaspoon dry mustard
2 tablespoons chopped ham
1 small sweet pickle, chopped
1 tablespoon chopped fresh parsley

In a saucepan, cover eggs with cold water; bring to a simmer. Gently simmer eggs about 11 or 12 minutes. Remove from heat and drain; cover with cold water and cool about 10 minutes. Crack and shell eggs. Cut eggs in half and remove yolks; discard 2 yolks. Mash remaining yolks in a small bowl and blend in remaining ingredients. Spoon mixture into egg cavities. Cover and refrigerate until needed. Makes 12 stuffed eggs.

Each half contains:

Cal.	Cal. from Fat	Protein	Carb.	Total Fiber	Total Fat	Sat. Fat	Chol.	Sodium
50	25	4g	2g	0g	3g	1g	109mg	104mg

Exchanges:

1/2 Medium Meat/Protein

Chile-Cheese Cakes

Add a green salad to this southwestern snack for a light lunch. Corn cakes may be found on the same grocery shelf as rice cakes.

1/4 cup (55 g) plain nonfat yogurt
1 green onion, chopped
1/4 teaspoon garlic powder
2 tablespoons chopped roasted peeled green chile
4 corn cakes
1 tomato, sliced
1/4 cup (30 g) shredded low-fat cheddar cheese

In a small bowl, combine yogurt, green onion, garlic powder and chile. Spread mixture evenly on top of corn cakes. Top with tomato slices and cheese. Place in microwave oven and cook on High until cheese melts. Serve at once. Makes 4 servings.

Each serving contains:

Cal.	Cal. from Fat	Protein	Carb.	Total Fiber	Total Fat	Sat. Fat	Chol.	Sodium
72	18	4g	10g	1g	2g	1g	11mg	98mg

Exchanges:

1 Bread/Starch, 1/2 Lean Meat/Protein

Breakfast & Brunch

Everyone should start the day with a nourishing breakfast, especially those with diabetes. This can be a meal to look forward to, even if you have been indifferent to breakfast in the past. Those who love lavish, but perhaps less healthful, breakfasts can find ways to enjoy the meal while also cutting back on fat and calories. The recipes in this section can help.

For those who like to sleep in and who may be short on time in the morning, try a Strawberry-Banana or Pineapple Smoothie. Let your blender do all the work—then pour your breakfast into a drink container and be on your way in record time.

If you prefer a cold breakfast, make your own Granola. Make a double batch and you will always have some available. If you love fruit as much as I do, you'll find that Fruit & Cottage Cheese Parfait is a cool and refreshing repast at any time of year.

For those who enjoy a more substantial, hot meal, fix Ranch-Style Eggs or a Spanish Omelet. Any of the pancake recipes are sure to be a hit, especially the Ginger-Pear Puffed Pancake.

Preparing brunch for family and friends is an easy way to entertain. Plan to serve something that is not everyday fare, such as Spinach Quiche and Apple-Poppy Seed Muffins, along with a colorful selection of fresh fruit.

Lots of us regularly eat breakfast out, in restaurants and coffee shops. Eating breakfast in a restaurant can pose a problem, because so many menus contain dishes that are high in fat and calories. A couple of tips can help you bring those high-fat, high-calorie meals into line. Start by making some simple substitutions for the heavier items, such as bacon and eggs, that you used to order. Try cottage cheese mixed with fresh fruit, or fresh fruit mixed with yogurt, for a filling and healthful way to start the day. A side order of fruit is also tasty as a sweet topping on hot or cold cereal. Instead of ordering a cheese Danish, try a dry toasted bagel and add a tablespoon of marmalade or strawberry jam as a spread.

Denver Scramble

For variety, serve this in a split pita pocket or wrap it in a flour tortilla.

1/4 onion, chopped
1 celery stalk
1/4 green bell pepper
2 eggs
2 egg whites
1/4 teaspoon dried leaf basil or parsley
Chili powder to taste

Spray a nonstick skillet with vegetable cooking spray. Heat skillet and add onion, celery and bell pepper. Sauté until softened. Add eggs, egg whites and basil or parsley to skillet. Stir quickly, moving all uncooked areas, until eggs are done as desired. Sprinkle with chili powder. Makes 4 servings.

Each serving contains:

Cal.	Cal. from Fat	Protein	Carb.	Total Fiber	Total Fat	Sat. Fat	Chol.	Sodium
52	23	5g	2g	0g	3g	1g	106mg	68mg

Exchanges:

1 Lean Meat/Protein, 1/2 Vegetable

Ranch-Style Eggs

A favorite breakfast or light supper dish in the Southwest, where it is known as huevos rancheros.

2 teaspoons canola oil
1/4 onion, chopped (about 2 tablespoons)
1 garlic clove, minced
2 roasted green chiles, peeled and chopped
3 tomatoes, chopped
2 tablespoons chopped fresh cilantro
1 teaspoon dried leaf oregano
4 eggs
4 corn tortillas
1/4 cup (30 g) reduced-fat cheddar cheese

Heat oil in a medium skillet. Add onion and garlic; sauté until softened, not browned. Stir in chiles, tomatoes, cilantro and oregano; cover and cook about 3 minutes. Break eggs into hot mixture; do not stir. Cover and cook as desired. Warm tortillas in a toaster oven or microwave. Place a tortilla on each plate; carefully spoon some of the tomato mixture on top. Place an egg on mixture and spoon remaining mixture around edge of tortilla. Sprinkle with cheese and serve at once. If desired, place dish under a broiler until cheese bubbles. Makes 4 servings.

Each serving contains:

Cal.	Cal. from Fat	Protein	Carb.	Total Fiber	Total Fat	Sat. Fat	Chol.	Sodium
198	79	11g	20g	3g	9g	2g	214mg	159mg

Exchanges:

1 Bread/Starch, 1 1/2 Lean Meat/Protein, 1 Vegetable, 1 Fat

Spanish Omelet

For those who prefer a mild filling with colorful eye appeal.

2 teaspoons olive oil
2 green onions, chopped
1/4 roasted red bell pepper, chopped
4 ounces (115 g) low-sodium ham, chopped
1 cup (250 ml) egg substitute
1/2 teaspoon ground cumin
1/4 teaspoon garlic powder
Paprika to taste

Heat oil in a medium skillet. Add green onions, bell pepper and ham; sauté until onions and pepper are softened. Pour in egg substitute; add cumin and garlic powder. Swirl egg mixture in skillet, lifting at edges to allow uncooked portion to flow under. Continue swirling until cooked as desired. Fold in half, cut into wedges, and sprinkle with paprika. Makes 4 servings.

Each serving contains:

Cal.	Cal. from Fat	Protein	Carb.	Total Fiber	Total Fat	Sat. Fat	Chol.	Sodium
125	60	14	2g	0g	6g	1g	16g	387mg

Exchanges:

2 Lean Meat/Protein, 1 Vegetable

Spinach Quiche

A classic brunch dish, excellent whether served hot or at room temperature.

1 (10-ounce/280-g) package frozen spinach
1 cup (230 g) plain nonfat yogurt
1 cup (230 g) nonfat cottage cheese
1 cup (250 ml) egg substitute
1/4 cup (30 g) shredded low-sodium Parmesan cheese
1/4 cup (30 g) crumbled feta cheese
1 tablespoon chopped sun-dried tomatoes
1 green onion, chopped
1/4 teaspoon dried leaf oregano
1/4 teaspoon ground nutmeg

Preheat oven to 350F (175C). Thaw spinach and place in a sieve. Squeeze excess water out of leaves before using. Place all ingredients in a food processor and blend. Pour mixture into 9-inch (23-cm) pie pan and bake 45 minutes. Serve hot or cold. Makes 6 servings.

Each serving contains:

Cal.	Cal. from Fat	Protein	Carb.	Total Fiber	Total Fat	Sat. Fat	Chol.	Sodium
129	28	16g	8g	2g	4g	2g	13mg	331mg

Exchanges:

1 1/2 Lean Meat/Protein, 1 Vegetable, 1/2 Skim Milk

Fruit & Cottage Cheese Parfait

Here is a great no-cook way to start the day; vary the fruit with the season.

1 cup (230 g) nonfat cottage cheese
1/4 cup (35 g) fresh blueberries
1 large apple, cored and chopped
2 tablespoons chopped walnuts

In a parfait glass or glass bowl, spoon alternating layers of cottage cheese and fruit. Top with chopped walnuts. Makes 2 servings.

Each serving contains:

Cal.	Cal. from Fat	Protein	Carb.	Total Fiber	Total Fat	Sat. Fat	Chol.	Sodium
200	42	17g	24g	4g	5g	0g	10mg	37mg

Exchanges:

2 Very Lean Meat/Protein, 1½ Fruit, 1 Fat

Granola

This crunchy mixture can be enjoyed in many ways, as a breakfast cereal, as a snack, or as a topping on fruit or yogurt.

2 cups (160 g) old-fashioned rolled oats
1 cup (30 g) wheat flakes
1/4 cup (20 g) unsweetened flaked coconut
1/4 cup (30 g) sliced almonds
1/4 cup (30 g) dried currants
1/4 cup (30 g) chopped dried apricots
1/4 cup (60 ml) honey
1/4 cup (60 ml) canola oil
1/2 teaspoon vanilla extract

Preheat oven to 325F (165C). Line a 13 x 9-inch (33 x 23-cm) baking pan with foil. In a large bowl, combine oats, wheat flakes, coconut, almonds, currants and apricots. In a cup, blend honey, oil and vanilla. Drizzle over dry mixture and stir to coat. Spread mixture evenly in baking pan. Bake 15 to 20 minutes, stirring several times until toasted. Cool and store in a covered container. Makes 8 servings.

Each serving contains:

Cal.	Cal. from Fat	Protein	Carb.	Total Fiber	Total Fat	Sat. Fat	Chol.	Sodium
268	99	6g	38g	5g	11g	2g	0mg	3mg

Exchanges:

2 Bread/Starch, 1/2 Fruit, 2 Fat

Cornmeal Rolls

Warm rolls add a special touch to any meal, and this no-yeast, no-rise version bakes in no time.

1/2 cup (85 g) cornmeal
1 1/2 cups (310 g) all-purpose flour
2 tablespoons sugar
2 teaspoons baking powder
1/2 teaspoon baking soda
1/4 teaspoon salt
1/4 cup (60) egg substitute
3/4 cup (170 g) plain nonfat yogurt

Preheat oven to 425F (220C). In a medium mixing bowl, combine cornmeal, flour, sugar, baking powder, baking soda and salt. Add egg substitute and yogurt. Stir together to make a soft dough. Roll out to a 1/4-inch (6-mm) thickness. Cut out 2-inch (5-cm) rounds. Fold each round in half. Bake on an ungreased baking sheet 15 minutes or until lightly browned. Makes about 24 rolls.

Each roll contains:

Cal.	Cal. from Fat	Protein	Carb.	Total Fiber	Total Fat	Sat. Fat	Chol.	Sodium
49	2	2g	10g	0g	0g	0g	0mg	79mg

Exchanges:

1 Bread/Starch

Apple-Poppy Seed Muffins

Fresh apple bits add extra moistness.

1¼ cups (175 g) all-purpose flour
3/4 cup (115 g) whole wheat flour
1/4 cup (55 g) sugar
1 tablespoon baking powder
1/2 teaspoon baking soda
1/2 cup (60 g) chopped fresh apple
1 tablespoon poppy seeds
1/2 cup (120 ml) egg substitute
1 cup (230 g) plain nonfat yogurt
3 tablespoons canola oil
1 teaspoon vanilla extract

Preheat oven to 400F (200C). Spray a 12-muffin pan with vegetable cooking spray or line with paper cups. In a bowl, stir together all-purpose flour, whole-wheat flour, sugar, baking powder, baking soda, apple and poppy seeds. Make a well in center of mixture and pour in egg substitute, yogurt, oil and vanilla. Mix together lightly until ingredients are moistened. Do not overmix. Spoon into prepared muffin pan. Bake about 20 minutes. Cool slightly before serving. Makes 12 muffins.

Each muffin contains:

Cal.	Cal. from Fat	Protein	Carb.	Total Fiber	Total Fat	Sat. Fat	Chol.	Sodium
144	39	5g	22g	1g	4g	0g	1mg	14mg

Exchanges:

1½ Bread/Starch, 1/2 Very Lean Meat/Protein, 1 Fat

Apricot Bran Muffins

Muffins made with bran will not rise as much as others.

1 cup (250 ml) reduced-fat buttermilk
1/4 cup (60 ml) egg substitute
3 tablespoons canola oil
1/3 cup (80 ml) molasses
1 1/2 cups (108 g) unprocessed bran
1/3 cup (55 g) chopped dried apricots
1/2 cup (70 g) all-purpose flour
1/4 cup (57 g) fructose granules
1 tablespoon baking powder
1 teaspoon baking soda

Preheat oven to 400F (200C). Spray a 12-muffin pan with vegetable cooking spray or line with paper cups. In a bowl, stir together buttermilk, egg substitute, oil and molasses. Add bran and apricots; mix and let stand at least 5 minutes. Add remaining ingredients and mix together lightly until ingredients are moistened. Do not overmix. Spoon into prepared muffin pan. Bake about 20 minutes. Cool slightly before serving. Makes 12 muffins.

Each muffin contains:

Cal.	Cal. from Fat	Protein	Carb.	Total Fiber	Total Fat	Sat. Fat	Chol.	Sodium
112	34	2g	18g	0g	4g	0g	1mg	197mg

Exchanges:

1 Bread/Starch, 1 Fat

Ginger-Pear Puffed Pancake

Serve at once while it is beautifully puffed.

2 tablespoons margarine
1 or 2 firm, ripe Anjou or bosc pears, cored and sliced
2/3 cup (95 g) all-purpose flour
2/3 cup (160 ml) fat- free milk
2 tablespoons sugar
1/4 cup (60 ml) orange juice
4 teaspoons chopped crystallized ginger
1/4 teaspoon ground cinnamon
2 eggs
2 egg whites

Preheat oven to 425F (220C). Melt margarine in a 9-inch (23-cm) deep-dish pie pan or quiche pan. Place pear slices in margarine, turning to coat all sides. Arrange slices in a pinwheel design in bottom of pan. In a bowl, blender, or food processor, combine remaining ingredients except egg whites; blend thoroughly. Beat egg whites until stiff peaks form and fold into mixture; carefully pour over pear slices. Bake 20 to 25 minutes or until golden brown and puffed. Most of the puffing occurs in the last 5 to 7 minutes. Serve at once. Makes 6 servings.

Each serving contains:

Cal.	Cal. from Fat	Protein	Carb.	Total Fiber	Total Fat	Sat. Fat	Chol.	Sodium
226	46	6g	40g	2g	5g	1g	71mg	109mg

Exchanges:

2 Bread/Starch, 1 Very Lean Meat/Protein, 1 Fruit, 1 Fat

Oatmeal Pancakes

For a change, top your pancakes with stewed apples or fresh fruit instead of syrup.

1/2 cup (40 g) old-fashioned rolled oats
1¼ cups (300 ml) reduced-fat buttermilk
1/4 cup (60 ml) egg substitute, or 2 egg whites, lightly beaten
1/2 cup (70 g) all-purpose flour
1/2 cup (70 g) whole wheat flour
1 tablespoon baking powder
1 teaspoon baking soda
1 teaspoon vanilla extract

Put oats in a medium mixing bowl and pour in buttermilk; stir and let stand 15 minutes. Beat in egg substitute or egg whites and remaining ingredients until well blended. Preheat a nonstick griddle. Spoon about 1/4 cup (60 ml) batter for each pancake. Cook pancakes until bubbles appear and edges look slightly dry. Turn and continue cooking until lightly browned. Makes 12 (3-inch) pancakes.

Each pancake contains:

Cal.	Cal. from Fat	Protein	Carb.	Total Fiber	Total Fat	Sat. Fat	Chol.	Sodium
65	7	3g	11g	1g	1g	0g	1mg	199mg

Exchanges:

1 Bread/Starch

Pistachio Pancakes

Tender pancakes are studded with delicious green pistachios.

1 cup (140 g) all-purpose flour
2 tablespoons brown sugar
1 tablespoon baking powder
1½ teaspoons baking soda
1 cup (250 ml) reduced-fat buttermilk
1 teaspoon vanilla extract
2 tablespoons canola oil
2 egg whites, lightly beaten
3 tablespoons chopped pistachios

Preheat a large nonstick skillet or griddle. Stir together flour, brown sugar, baking powder and baking soda in a medium mixing bowl. Beat in buttermilk, vanilla, oil and egg whites. Add chopped pistachios. Lightly spray skillet or griddle with vegetable cooking spray. Pour 1/4 cup (60 ml) batter for each pancake. Cook 2 to 3 minutes or until bubbles appear and surface looks dry. Turn; cook 2 to 3 minutes, until browned. Makes 12 (3-inch) pancakes.

Each pancake contains:

Cal.	Cal. from Fat	Protein	Carb.	Total Fiber	Total Fat	Sat. Fat	Chol.	Sodium
272	95	8g	36g	1g	11g	1g	2mg	582mg

Exchanges:

2 Bread/Starch, 1 Very Lean Meat/Protein, 2 Fat

Spicy Baked French Toast

This dish can be prepared the night before or several hours ahead. Be sure to cover and refrigerate it until baking time.

1 cup (250 ml) egg substitute
1 cup (250 ml) fat-free milk
1 tablespoon sugar
1/2 teaspoon ground cinnamon
1/4 teaspoon ground nutmeg
1/4 teaspoon ground allspice
1/2 teaspoon almond extract
8 slices white bread

Preheat oven to 400F (200C). Line a baking sheet with foil and spray with vegetable cooking spray. In a shallow dish, combine egg substitute, milk, sugar, cinnamon, nutmeg, allspice and almond extract. Dip bread into mixture, turning to coat both sides; place on prepared baking sheet. Cover with foil or plastic wrap and let stand about 20 minutes. Uncover and bake about 10 minutes; turn slices over and bake another 5 minutes. Serve at once. Makes 4 servings.

Each 2-slice serving contains:

Cal.	Cal. from Fat	Protein	Carb.	Total Fiber	Total Fat	Sat. Fat	Chol.	Sodium
250	39	15g	36g	2g	4g	1g	2mg	466mg

Exchanges:

2½ Bread/Starch, 2 Very Lean Meat/Protein, 1 Fat

Buttermilk Pecan Waffles

Chocolate and pecans—what a heavenly combination for special weekend waffles!

- **1½ cups (215 g) all-purpose flour**
- **2 tablespoons unsweetened cocoa powder**
- **2 teaspoons baking powder**
- **1 teaspoon baking soda**
- **2 teaspoons sugar**
- **3 tablespoons chopped pecans**
- **1¼ cups (300 ml) reduced-fat buttermilk**
- **3 tablespoons canola oil**
- **3 egg whites, beaten lightly**

Preheat waffle maker. In a bowl, stir together flour, cocoa powder, baking powder, baking soda, sugar and pecans. Mix in buttermilk and oil. Fold in egg whites. Bake according to manufacturer's instructions. Makes 6 (6-inch) waffles.

Each waffle contains:

Cal.	Cal. from Fat	Protein	Carb.	Total Fiber	Total Fat	Sat. Fat	Chol.	Sodium
238	93	7g	30g	2g	10g	1g	2mg	368mg

Exchanges:

2 Bread/Starch, 1 Very Lean Meat/Protein, 2 Fat

Strawberry-Banana Smoothie

Delicious not just for breakfast but for any time you need a lift.

1 small banana
1/2 cup (115 g) plain nonfat yogurt
1/2 cup (120 ml) fat-free milk
1 cup (150 g) sliced strawberries
3 ice cubes

Combine all ingredients in a blender or food processor. Purée until mixture is smooth. Makes 2 (10-ounce) servings.

Each serving contains:

Cal.	Cal. from Fat	Protein	Carb.	Total Fiber	Total Fat	Sat. Fat	Chol.	Sodium
118	6	6g	25g	3g	1g	0g	2mg	68mg

Exchanges:

1½ Fruit, 1/2 Skim Milk

Pineapple Smoothie

Tropical fruits have a natural sweetness that makes additional sugar unnecessary.

1 (8-ounce/230-g) can juice-packed pineapple chunks
1/4 cup (60 ml) pineapple juice from can
1/2 cup (115 g) plain nonfat yogurt
1/4 cup (60 ml) evaporated skimmed milk
1/2 banana
3 ice cubes

Combine all ingredients in a blender. Purée until mixture is smooth. Makes 2 (8-ounce) servings.

Each serving contains:

Cal.	Cal. from Fat	Protein	Carb.	Total Fiber	Total Fat	Sat. Fat	Chol.	Sodium
150	6	6g	34g	2g	1g	0g	2mg	73mg

Exchanges:

2 Fruit, 1/2 Skim Milk

Cucumber-Mint Smoothie

A refreshing, light drink that is a perfect accompaniment to brunch or Middle Eastern cuisine.

1½ cups (170 g) seeded and chopped cucumber
1/2 cup (115 g) plain nonfat yogurt
1/2 cup ice
6 fresh mint leaves
1/4 cup (60 ml) evaporated skimmed milk
1 teaspoon grated lemon zest
Salt and black pepper to taste

Combine ingredients in a blender. Purée until mixture is smooth. Makes 4 (6-ounce) servings.

Each serving contains:

Cal.	Cal. from Fat	Protein	Carb.	Total Fiber	Total Fat	Sat. Fat	Chol.	Sodium
31	1	3g	5g	0g	0g	0g	1mg	37mg

Exchanges:

1/2 Skim Milk

Exchange Lists

Starch List

Cereals, grains, pasta, breads, crackers, snacks, starchy vegetables and cooked beans, peas and lentils are starches. In general, one starch is

- 1/2 cup of cereal, grain, pasta or starchy vegetable,
- 1 ounce of a bread product, such as 1 slice of bread.
- 3/4 to 1 ounce of most snack foods. (Some snack foods may also have added fat.)

One starch exchange equals
15 grams carbohydrate, 0-1 grams fat, 3 grams protein, 80 calories.

Bread

Bagel	1/2 (1 oz.)
Bread, reduced-calorie	2 slices (1½ oz.)
Bread, white, whole-wheat, pumpernickel, rye	1 slice (1 oz.)
Bread sticks, crisp, 4 in. long x 1/2 in.	2 (2/3 oz.)
English muffin	1/2
Hot dog or hamburger bun	1/2 (1 oz.)
Pita, 6 in. across	1/2
Roll, plain, small	1 (1 oz.)
Raisin bread, unfrosted	1 slice (1 oz.)
Tortilla, corn, 6 in. across	1
Tortilla, flour, 6 in. across	1
Waffle, 4½ in. square, reduced-fat	1

Cereals and Grains

Bran cereals	1/2 cup
Bulgur	1/2 cup
Cereals	1/2 cup
Cereals, unsweetened, ready-to-eat	3/4 cup
Cornmeal (dry)	3 tablespoons
Couscous	1/3 cup
Flour (dry)	3 tablespoons
Granola, low-fat	1/4 cup
Grape-Nuts	1/4 cup
Grits	1/2 cup
Kasha	1/2 cup
Millet	1/4 cup
Muesli	1/4 cup
Oats	1/2 cup
Pasta	1/2 cup
Puffed cereal	1½ cups
Rice milk	1/2 cup
Rice, white or brown	1/3 cup
Shredded Wheat®	1/2 cup
Sugar-frosted cereal	1/2 cup
Wheat germ	3 tablespoons

American Dietetic Association
The Exchange Lists are the basis of a meal planning system designed by a committee of the American Diabetes Association and The American Dietetic Association. While designed primarily for people with diabetes and others who must follow special diets, the Exchange Lists are based on principles of good nutrition that apply to everyone.
© 1995 American Diabetes Association, Inc., The American Dietetic Association. Used by permission.

Starchy Vegetables

Baked beans . . . . .1/3 cup
Corn . . . . .1/2 cup
Corn on cob, medium . . . . . .1 (5 oz.)
Mixed vegetables with
    corn, peas or pasta . . . . .1 cup
Peas, green . . . . .1/2 cup
Plantain . . . . .1/2 cup
Potato, baked or boiled . . . . . .1 small
(3 oz.)
Potato, mashed . . . . .1/2 cup
Squash, winter . . . . .1 cup
    (acorn, butternut, pumpkin)
Yam, sweet potato, plain . . . .1/2 cup

Crackers and Snacks

Animal crackers 8
Graham crackers, 2 1/2 in. square . .3
Matzoh . . . . .3/4 oz.
Melba toast . . . . .4 slices
Oyster crackers 24
Popcorn . . . . .3 cups
    (popped, no fat added or
    low-fat microwave)
Pretzels . . . . .3/4 oz.
Rice cakes, 4 in. across 2
Saltine-type crackers 6
Snack chips, fat-free . .15-20 (3/4 oz.)
    (tortilla, potato)
Whole-wheat crackers,
    no fat added . . . . .2-5 (3/4 oz.)

Beans, Peas and Lentils
Count as 1 starch exchange, plus
1 very lean meat exchange

Beans and peas . . . . .1/2 cup
    (garbanzo, pinto, kidney,
    white, split, black-eyed)
Lima beans . . . . .2/3 cup
Lentils . . . . .1/2 cup
Miso* . . . . .3 tablespoons

Starchy Foods Prepared with Fat
Count as 1 starch exchange, plus
1 fat exchange

Biscuit, 2 1/2 in. across 1
Chow mein noodles . . . . .1/2 cup
Corn bread, 2-in. cube . . . . . .1 (2 oz.)
Crackers, round butter type 6
Croutons . . . . .1 cup
French-fried potatoes . . .16-25 (3 oz.)
Granola . . . . .1/4 cup
Muffin, small . . . . .1 (1 1/2 oz.)
Pancake, 4 in. across 2
Popcorn, microwave . . . . . . .3 cups
Sandwich crackers, cheese or
    peanut butter filling 3
Stuffing, bread (prepared) . . .1/3 cup
Taco shell, 6 in. across 2
Waffle, 4 1/2 in. square 1
Whole-wheat crackers,
    fat added . . . . .4-6 (1 oz.)

Fruit List

Fresh, frozen, canned and dried fruits and fruit juices are on this list. In general, one fruit exchange equals

- 1 small to medium fresh fruit
- 1/2 cup of canned or fresh fruit juice
- 1/4 cup of dried fruit

One fruit exchange equals
15 grams carbohydrate and 60 calories.
The weight includes skin, core, seeds and rind.

---

* = 400 mg or more sodium per exchange.

Fruit

Apple, unpeeled, small . . . . .1 (4 oz.)
Applesauce, unsweetened . . .1/2 cup
Apples, dried . . . . .4 rings
Apricots, fresh . . . . .4 whole (5½ oz.)
Apricots, dried . . . . .8 halves
Apricots, canned . . . . .1/2 cup
Banana, small . . . . .1 (4 oz.)
Blackberries . . . . .3/4 cup
Blueberries . . . . .3/4 cup
Cantaloupe, small . . . . .1/3 melon
(11 oz.) or 1 cup cubes
Cherries, sweet, fresh . . . . .12 (3 oz.)
Cherries, sweet, canned . . . . .1/2 cup
Dates 3
Figs, fresh . . . .1½ large or 2 medium
(3½ oz.)
Figs, dried 1½
Fruit cocktail . . . . .1/2 cup
Grapefruit, large . . . . .1/2 (11 oz.)
Grapefruit sections, canned . .3/4 cup
Grapes, small . . . . .17 (3 oz.)
Honeydew melon . . . .1 slice (10 oz.)
or 1 cup cubes
Kiwi . . . . .1 (3½ oz.)
Mandarin oranges, canned . . 3/4 cup
Mango, small . . . . .1/2 fruit
(5½ oz.) or 1/2 cup
Nectarine, small . . . . .1 (5 oz.)
Orange, small . . . . .1 (6½ oz.)

Papaya . . . . .1/2 fruit (8 oz.)
or 1 cup cubes
Peach, medium, fresh . . . . . .1 (6 oz.)
Peaches,canned . . . . .1/2 cup
Pear, large, fresh . . . . .1/2 (4 oz.)
Pears, canned . . . . .1/2 cup
Pineapple, fresh . . . . .3/4 cup
Pineapple, canned . . . . .1/2 cup
Plums, small . . . . .2 (5 oz.)
Plums, canned . . . . .1/2 cup
Prunes, dried 3
Raisins . . . . .2 tablespoons
Raspberries . . . . .1 cup
Strawberries . . .1¼ cups whole berries
Tangerines, small . . . . .2 (8 oz.)
Watermelon . . . . . . .1 slice (13½ oz.)
or 1¼ cup cubes

Fruit Juice

Apple juice/cider . . . . .1/2 cup
Cranberry juice cocktail . . . . . .1/3 cup
Cranberry juice cocktail,
reduced-calorie . . . . .1 cup
Fruit juice blends,
100% juice . . . . .1/3 cup
Grape juice . . . . .1/3 cup
Grapefruit juice . . . . .1/2 cup
Orange juice . . . . .1/2 cup
Pineapple juice . . . . .1/2 cup
Prune juice . . . . .1/3 cup

Milk List

Different types of milk and milk products are on this list. Cheeses are on the Meat list and cream and other dairy fats are on the Fat list. Based on the amount of fat they contain, milks are divided into fat-free/low-fat milk, reduced-fat milk and whole milk. One choice of these includes

	Carbohydrate (grams)	Protein (grams)	Fat (grams)	Calories
Fat-free/low-fat	12	8	0-3	90
Reduced-fat	12	8	5	120
Whole	12	8	8	150

One milk exchange equals
12 grams carbohydrate and 8 grams protein.

Fat-Free and Low-Fat Milk
0-3 grams fat per serving

Fat-free milk . . . . .1 cup
1/2% milk . . . . .1 cup
1% milk . . . . .1 cup
Fat-free or low-fat buttermilk . . .1 cup
Evaporated fat-free milk . . . . .1/2 cup
Fat-free dry milk . . . . .1/3 cup dry
Plain nonfat yogurt . . . . .3/4 cup
Nonfat or low-fat fruit-
  flavored yogurt sweetened
  with aspartame or with a
  non-nutritive sweetener . . . . . .1 cup

Reduced-Fat
5 grams fat per serving

2% milk . . . . .1 cup
Plain low-fat yogurt . . . . . . .3/4 cup
Sweet acidophilus milk . . . . . . .1 cup

Whole Milk
8 grams fat per serving

Whole milk . . . . .1 cup
Evaporated whole milk . . . . . .1/2 cup
Goat's milk . . . . .1 cup
Kefir .1 cup

Other Carbohydrates List

You can substitute food choices from this list for a starch, fruit, or milk choice on your meal plan. Some choices will also count as one or more fat choices.

One exchange equals
15 grams carbohydrate, or 1 starch, or 1 fruit, or 1 milk.

Food	Serving Size	Exchanges per Serving
Angel food cake, unfrosted	1/12th cake	2 carbohydrates
Brownie, small, unfrosted	2 in. square	1 carbohydrate, 1 fat
Cake, unfrosted	2 in. square	1 carbohydrate, 1 fat
Cake, frosted	2 in. square	2 carbohydrates, 1 fat
Cookie, fat-free	2 small	1 carbohydrate
Cookie or sandwich cookie with creme filling	2 small	1 carbohydrate, 1 fat
Cranberry sauce, jellied	1/4 cup	1 1/2 carbohydrates
Cupcake, frosted	1 small	2 carbohydrates, 1 fat
Doughnut, plain cake	1 medium (1 1/2 oz.)	1 1/2 carbs, 2 fats
Doughnut, glazed	3 1/2 in. across (2 oz.)	2 carbohydrates, 2 fats
Fruit juice bars, frozen, 100% juice	1 bar (3 oz.)	1 carbohydrate
Fruit snacks, chewy (puréed fruit concentrate)	1 roll (3/4 oz.)	1 carbohydrate
Fruit spreads, 100% fruit	1 tablespoon	1 carbohydrate
Gelatin, regular	1/2 cup	1 carbohydrate
Gingersnaps	3	1 carbohydrate
Granola bar	1 bar	1 carbohydrate, 1 fat
Granola bar, fat-free	1 bar	2 carbohydrates
Honey	1 tablespoon	1 carbohydrate
Hummus	1/3 cup	1 carbohydrate, 1 fat
Ice cream	1/2 cup	1 carbohydrate, 2 fats
Ice cream, light	1/2 cup	1 carbohydrate, 1 fat
Ice cream, fat-free, no sugar added	1/2 cup	1 carbohydrate
Jam or jelly, regular	1 tablespoon	1 carbohydrate
Milk, chocolate, whole	1 cup	2 carbohydrates, 1 fat

One exchange equals
15 grams carbohydrate, or 1 starch, or 1 fruit, or 1 milk

Food	Serving Size	Exchanges per Serving
Pie, fruit, 2 crusts	1/6 pie	3 carbohydrates, 2 fats
Pie, pumpkin or custard	1/8 pie	2 carbohydrates, 2 fats
Potato chips	12-18 (1 oz.)	1 carbohydrate, 2 fats
Pudding, regular (made with low-fat milk)	1/2 cup	2 carbohydrates
Pudding, sugar-free (made with low-fat milk)	1/2 cup	1 carbohydrate
Salad dressing, fat-free*	1/4 cup	1 carbohydrate
Sherbet, sorbet	1/2 cup	2 carbohydrates
Spaghetti or pasta sauce, canned*	1/2 cup	1 carbohydrate, 1 fat
Sugar	1 tablespoon	1 carbohydrate
Sweet roll or Danish	1 (2½ oz.)	2½ carbohydrates, 2 fats
Syrup, light	2 tablespoons	1 carbohydrate
Syrup, regular	1 tablespoon	1 carbohydrate
Syrup, regular	1/4 cup	4 carbohydrates
Tortilla chips	6-12 (1 oz.)	1 carbohydrate, 2 fats
Vanilla wafers	5	1 carbohydrate, 1 fat
Yogurt, frozen, low-fat, fat-free	1/3 cup	1 carbohydrate, 0-1 fat
Yogurt, frozen, fat-free, no sugar added	1/2 cup	1 carbohydrate
Yogurt, low-fat with fruit	1 cup	3 carbohydrates, 0-1 fat

Vegetable List

Vegetables that contain small amounts of carbohydrates and calories are on this list. Vegetables contain important nutrients. Try to eat at least 2 or 3 vegetable choices each day. In general, one vegetable exchange is

- 1/2 cup of cooked vegetables or vegetable juice
- 1 cup raw vegetables
- If you eat 1 or 2 vegetable choices at a meal or snack, you do not have to count the calories or carbohydrates because they contain small amounts of these nutrients.

One vegetable exchange equals
5 grams carbohydrate, 0 grams fat, 2 grams protein, 25 calories.

Artichoke	Beets	Celery
Artichoke hearts	Broccoli	Cucumber
Asparagus	Brussels sprouts	Eggplant
Beans (green, wax, Italian)	Cabbage	Green onions or scallions
Bean sprouts	Carrots	Greens (collard, kale, mustard, turnip)
	Cauliflower	

* = 400 mg or more sodium per exchange.

Kohlrabi

Leeks

Mixed vegetables
(without corn, peas,
or pasta)

Mushrooms

Okra

Onions

Pea pods

Peppers (all varieties)

Radishes

Salad greens (endive,
escarole, lettuce,
romaine, spinach)

Sauerkraut*

Spinach

Summer squash

Tomato

Tomatoes, canned

Tomato sauce*

Tomato/vegetable juice*

Turnips

Water chestnuts

Watercress

Zucchini

Meat and Meat Substitutes List

Meat and meat substitutes that contain both protein and fat are on this list. In general, one meat exchange is

- 1 oz. meat, fish, poultry, or cheese
- 1/2 cup beans, peas, and lentils
- Based on the amount of fat they contain, meats are divided into very lean, lean, medium-fat and high-fat lists. This is done so you can see which contain the least amount of fat. One ounce (one exchange) of each of these includes

	Carbohydrate (grams)	Protein (grams)	Fat (grams)	Calories
Very lean	0	7	0-1	35
Lean	0	7	3	55
Medium-fat	0	7	5	75
High-fat	0	7	8	100

Very Lean Meat and Substitutes
One exchange equals 0 grams carbohydrate, 7 grams protein, 0-1 grams fat and 35 calories.

- One very lean meat exchange is equal to any one of the following items.

Poultry: Chicken or turkey (white meat, no skin), Cornish hen (no skin) . . . . .1 oz.

Fish: Fresh or frozen cod, flounder, haddock, halibut, trout; tuna fresh or canned in water . . . . .1 oz.

Shellfish: Clams, crab, lobster, scallops, shrimp, imitation shellfish . . . . .1 oz.

Game: Duck or pheasant (no skin), venison, buffalo, ostrich . . . . . .1 oz.

Cheese: (with 1 gram or less fat per ounce)
Nonfat or low-fat cottage cheese . . . . .1/4 cup
Fat-free cheese . . . . .1 oz.

Other: Processed sandwich meats with 1 gram or less fat per ounce, such as deli thin, shaved meats, chipped beef*, turkey ham . . . . .1 oz.
Egg whites .2
Egg substitutes, plain . . . . . . .1/4 cup
Hot dogs with 1 gram or less fat per ounce* . . . . .1 oz.
Kidney (high in cholesterol) . . . . .1 oz.
Sausage with 1 gram or less fat per ounce . . . . .1 oz.

* = 400 mg or more sodium per exchange.

• Count as one very lean meat and one starch exchange.

Beans, peas, lentils (cooked) . .1/2 cup

Lean Meat and Substitutes List

One exchange equals 0 grams carbohydrate, 7 grams protein, 3 grams fat and 55 calories.

• One lean meat exchange is equal to any one of the following items.

Beef: USDA Select or Choice grades of lean trimmed of fat, such as round, sirloin, and flank steak; tenderloin; roast (rib, chuck, rump); steak (T-bone, porterhouse, cubed), ground round . . . . .1 oz.

Pork: Lean pork, such as fresh ham; canned, cured or boiled ham; Canadian bacon*; tenderloin, center loin chop . . .1 oz.

Lamb: Roast, chop, leg . . . . .1 oz.

Veal: Lean chop, roast . . . . .1 oz.

Poultry: Chicken, turkey (dark meat, no skin), chicken (white meat, with skin), domestic duck or goose (well-drained of fat, no skin) . . .1 oz.

Fish:
Herring (uncreamed or smoked) . . . . .1 oz.
Oysters . . . . .6 medium
Salmon (fresh or canned), catfish . . . . .1 oz.
Sardines (canned) . . . . . . .2 medium
Tuna (canned in oil, drained) . . .1 oz.

Game: Goose (no skin), rabbit . .1 oz.

Cheese:
4.5%-fat cottage cheese . . . .1/4 cup
Grated Parmesan . . . .2 tablespoons
Cheeses with 3 grams or less fat per ounce . . . . .1 oz.

Other:
Hot dogs with 3 grams or less fat per ounce* . . . . . . .1 1/2 oz.

Processed sandwich meat with 3 grams or less fat per ounce, such as turkey pastrami or kielbasa . . . . .1 oz.
Liver, heart (high in cholesterol) . . . . .1 oz.

Medium-Fat Meat and Substitutes List

One exchange equals 0 grams carbohydrate, 7 grams protein, 5 grams fat and 75 calories.

• One medium-fat meat exchange is equal to any one of the following items.

Beef: Most beef products fall into this category (ground beef, meatloaf, corned beef, short ribs, Prime grades of meat trimmed of fat, such as prime rib) . . . . . .1 oz.

Pork: Top loin, chop, Boston butt, cutlet . . . . .1 oz.

Lamb: Rib roast, ground . . . . . . .1 oz.

Veal: Cutlet (ground or cubed, unbreaded) . . . . .1 oz.

Poultry: Chicken (dark meat, with skin), ground turkey or ground chicken, fried chicken (with skin) . . . . .1 oz.

Fish: Any fried fish product . . . . .1 oz.

Cheese: (with 5 grams or less fat per ounce)
Feta .1 oz.
Mozzarella . . . . .1 oz.
Ricotta . . . . .1/4 cup (2 oz.)

Other:
Egg (high in cholesterol, limit to 3 per week) 1
Sausage with 5 grams or less fat per ounce . . . . .1 oz.
Soy milk . . . . .1 cup
Tempeh . . . . .1/4 cup
Tofu . . . . .4 oz. or 1/2 cup

* = 400 mg or more sodium per exchange.

High-Fat Meat and Substitutes List
One exchange equals 0 grams carbohydrate, 7 grams protein, 8 grams fat and 100 calories.

Remember these items are high in saturated fat, cholesterol and calories, and may raise blood cholesterol levels if eaten on a regular basis.

- One high-fat meat exchange is equal to any one of the following items.

Pork: Spareribs, ground pork, pork sausage . . . . .1 oz.

Cheese: All regular cheeses, such as American*, cheddar, Monterey Jack, Swiss . . . . .1 oz.

Other:
Processed sandwich meats with 8 grams or less fat per ounce, such as bologna, pimento loaf, salami . . . . .1 oz.

Sausage, such as bratwurst, Italian, knockwurst, Polish, smoked . . . . .1 oz.

Hot dog (turkey or chicken)* 1 (10/pound)

Bacon . . . . .3 slices (20 slices/pound)

- Count as one high-fat meat plus one fat exchange.

Hot dog (beef, pork or combination)* 1 (10/pound)

- Count as one high-fat meat plus two fat exchanges.

Peanut butter (contains unsaturated fat) . . . . .2 tablespoons

Fat List

Fats are divided into three groups, based on the main type of fat they contain: monounsaturated, polyunsaturated and saturated. Small amounts of monounsaturated and polyunsaturated fats in the foods we eat are linked with good health benefits. Saturated fats are linked with heart disease and cancer. In general, one fat exchange is

- 1 teaspoon of regular margarine or vegetable oil
- 1 tablespoon of regular salad dressings

Monounsaturated Fats List
One fat exchange equals 5 grams fat and 45 calories.

Avocado, medium . . . . .1/8 (1 oz.)

Oil (canola, olive, peanut) . . . . .1 teaspoon

Olives, ripe (black) . . . . .8 large
green, stuffed* . . . . .10 large

Nuts:
almonds, cashews . . . . .6 nuts
mixed (50% peanuts) . . . . . . .6 nuts
peanuts . . . . .10 nuts
pecans . . . . .4 halves

Peanut butter, smooth or crunchy . . . . .2 teaspoons

Sesame seeds . . . . .1 tablespoon

Tahini paste . . . . .2 teaspoons

* = 400 mg or more sodium per exchange.

Polyunsaturated Fats List
One fat exchange equals 5 grams fat and 45 calories.

Margarine, stick, tub, or squeeze . . . . .1 teaspoon
lower-fat (30 to 50% vegetable oil) . . . . .1 tablespoon

Mayonnaise, regular . . . . .1 teaspoon
reduced-fat . . . . .1 tablespoon

Nuts, walnuts, English . . . . . .4 halves

Oil (corn, safflower, soybean) . . . . .1 teaspoon

Salad dressing, regular* .1 tablespoon
reduced-fat . . . . .2 tablespoons

Miracle Whip® Salad Dressing*, regular . . . . .2 teaspoons
reduced-fat . . . . .1 tablespoon

Seeds, pumpkin, sunflower . . . . .1 tablespoon

Saturated Fats List**
One fat exchange equals
5 grams of fat.

Bacon, cooked . . . . .1 slice
(20 slices/pound)
Bacon, grease . . . . .1 teaspoon
Butter, stick . . . . .1 teaspoon
whipped . . . . .2 teaspoons
reduced-fat . . . . .1 tablespoon
Chitterlings, boiled . . . .2 tablespoons
(1/2 oz.)
Coconut, sweetened,
shredded . . . . .2 tablespoons
Cream, half-and-half . . .2 tablespoons
Cream cheese,
regular . . . . . .1 tablespoon (1/2 oz.)
reduced-fat . . .2 tablespoons (1 oz.)
Fatback or salt pork, see below***
Shortening or lard . . . . . . .1 teaspoon
Sour cream, regular . . . .2 tablespoons
reduced-fat . . . . .3 tablespoons

Free Foods List

A free food is any food or drink that contains fewer than 20 calories or less than 5 grams of carbohydrate per serving. Foods with a serving size listed should be limited to three servings per day. Be sure to spread them out throughout the day. If you eat all three servings at one time, it could affect your blood glucose level. Foods listed without a serving size can be eaten as often as you like.

Fat-Free or Reduced-Fat Foods

Cream cheese, fat-free . .1 tablespoon
Creamers, nondairy,
liquid . . . . .1 tablespoon
Creamers, nondairy,
powdered . . . . .2 teaspoons
Mayonnaise, fat-free . . .1 tablespoon
reduced-fat . . . . .1 teaspoon
Margarine, fat-free . . . .4 tablespoons
reduced-fat . . . . .1 teaspoon
Miracle Whip®, nonfat . .1 tablespoon
reduced-fat . . . . .1 teaspoon
Nonstick cooking spray
Salad dressing, fat-free . .1 tablespoon
fat-free, Italian . . . . . .2 tablespoons
Salsa . . . . .1/4 cup
Sour cream, fat-free,
reduced-fat . . . . .1 tablespoon
Whipped topping,
regular or light . . . . . .2 tablespoons

Sugar-Free or Low-Sugar Foods

Candy, hard, sugar-free . . . . . .1 piece

Gelatin dessert, sugar-free
Gelatin, unflavored
Gum, sugar-free
Jam or jelly, low-sugar
or light . . . . .2 teaspoons
Sugar substitutes[†]
Syrup, sugar-free . . . . . .2 tablespoons

Drinks

Bouillon, broth, consommé*
Bouillon or broth, low-sodium
Carbonated or mineral water
Club soda
Cocoa powder,
unsweetened . . . . .1 tablespoon
Coffee
Diet soft drinks, sugar-free
Drink mixes, sugar-free
Tea
Tonic water, sugar-free

---

* = 400 mg or more sodium per exchange.

**Saturated fats can raise blood cholesterol levels.

***Use a piece 1 in. x 1 in. x 1/4 in. if you plan to eat the fatback cooked with vegetables. Use a piece 2 in. x 1 in. when eating only the vegetables with the fatback removed.

[†]Sugar substitutes, alternatives or replacements that are approved by the Food and Drug Administration (FDA) are safe to use. Common brand names include Equal® (aspartame), Sprinkle Sweet® (saccharin), Sweet One® (acesulfame K), Sweet-10® (saccharin), Sugar Twin® (saccharin), Sweet 'n Low® (saccharin).

Condiments

Catsup . . . . .1 tablespoon
Horseradish
Lemon juice
Lime juice
Mustard

Pickles, dill* . . . . .1½ large
Soy sauce, regular
    or light* . . . . .1 tablespoon
Taco sauce . . . . .1 tablespoon
Vinegar

Fast Foods*

Food	Serving Size	Exchanges per Serving
Burritos with beef*	2	4 carbohydrates, 2 medium-fat meats, 2 fats
Chicken nuggets*	6	1 carbohydrate, 2 medium-fat meats, 1 fat
Chicken breast and wing, breaded and fried*	1 each	1 carbohydrate, 4 medium-fat meats, 2 fats
Fish sandwich/tartar sauce*	1	3 carbohydrates, 1 medium-fat meat, 3 fats
French fries, thin*	20-25	2 carbohydrates, 2 fats
Hamburger, regular	1	2 carbohydrates, 2 medium-fat meats
Hamburger, large*	1	2 carbohydrates, 3 medium-fat meats, 1 fat
Hot dog with bun*	1	1 carbohydrate, 1 high-fat meat, 1 fat
Individual pan pizza*	1	5 carbohydrates, 3 medium-fat meats, 3 fats
Soft-serve cone	1 medium	2 carbohydrates, 1 fat
Submarine sandwich*	1 sub (6 in.)	3 carbohydrates, 1 vegetable, 2 medium-fat meats, 1 fat
Taco, hard shell*	1 (6 oz.)	2 carbohydrates, 2 medium-fat meats, 2 fats
Taco, soft shell*	1 (3 oz.)	1 carbohydrate, 1 medium-fat meat, 1 fat

* = 400 mg or more sodium per exchange.

Bibliography

American Diabetes Association and The American Dietetic Association. *Exchange Lists for Meal Planning*, Revised, 1995.

American Diabetes Association. Position statement: Diabetes mellitus and exercise. *Diabetes Care* 23 Supplement 1, 2000.

_____. Position statement: Nutrition recommendations and principles for people with diabetes mellitus. *Diabetes Care* 23 Supplement 1, 2000.

Centers for Disease Control and Prevention. National Diabetes Fact Sheet: National estimates and general information on diabetes in the United States. Revised edition. Atlanta, Georgia: U.S. Department of Health and Human Services, Centers for Disease Control and Prevention, 1998.

Chitwood, Marti. Botanical therapies for diabetes. *Diabetes Care and Education* 20, no. 6, 1999.

Expert Panel on Type 2 Diabetes in Adolescents and Children. *Pediatrics* 105:671-680, 2000.

O'Connell, Belinda. New Products Column: Butter, butter, butter . . . Parkay! A review of new margarines and low-fat spreads. *Diabetes Care and Education* 5, 1999.

U.S. Department of Health and Human Services, Public Health Service, Food and Drug Administration, and Center for Food Safety and Applied Nutrition. *A Food Labeling Guide*. 1994.

Web Sites

Centers for Disease Control
www.cdc.gov/diabetes/pub/facts98.htm

American Diabetes Association
www.diabetes.org
(800) 342-2383

American Dietetics Association
www.eatright.org
(800) 877-1600

Index